The Horn E

THE HORN BOOK

A GIRL'S GUIDE TO THE KNOWLEDGE OF GOOD AND EVIL

Anonymous

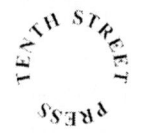

TENTH STREET PRESS

THIS EDITION

© Copyright 2015 Tenth Street Press

First published anonymously 1898
(As an adaptation of *Instruction Libertine*,
published in Paris, 1860)

ISBN10: 0-9942955-1-0
ISBN13: 978-0-9942955-1-4

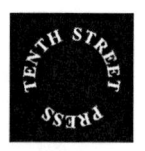

This book is sold on the condition that it shall not, by way of trade or otherwise, be lent, re-sold or circulated by any traditional or electronic means or have any original content contained herein reproduced in any form without prior written consent from the copyright holder.

TENTH STREET PRESS Ltd.
MELBOURNE LONDON
www.tenthstreetpress.com
Email: contact@tenthstreetpress.com

TABLE OF CONTENTS

INTRODUCTION   9

ENTRANCE TO THE TEMPLE

DIALOGUE I
ON THE PHYSICAL CONFORMATION OF
MAN AND WOMAN   15

THE SEXUAL PARTS OF MAN   20

THE SEXUAL PARTS OF WOMAN   23

DIALOGUE II
ON THE PLEASURES OF SOLITARY
MASTURBATION SODOMY AND TRIBADISM   33

MASCULINE SOLITARY MASTURBATION   38

FEMININE SOLITARY MASTURBATION   43

SODOMY, OR MAN WITH MAN   46

TRIBADISM, OR WOMEN WITH WOMEN   53

DIALOGUE III
ON THE VARIOUS WAYS OF VARYING THE
PLEASURES OF LOVE BETWEEN
MAN AND WOMAN   61

TABLE OF CONTENTS

CHAPTER I
POSTURES GIVING COMPLETE ENJOYMENT TO
TWO LOVERS 65

SECTION I
POSTURES WITH INTRODUCTION OF
THE MEMBER
INTRODUCTION OF THE COCK IN THE CUNT 66

DIALOGUE IV 107

DIALOGUE V

SODOMY WITH WOMEN 123

SECTION II
POSTURES WITHOUT INTRODUCTION OF THE
VIRIL MEMBER, BUT MUTUALLY VOLUPTUOUS;
RECIPROCAL FRIGGING AND GAMAHUCHING 129

CHAPTER II
PLEASURES OF MAN ALONE, BY THE AID OF
WOMAN, BUT WITHOUT HER RECIPROCAL
PARTICIPATION 143

CHAPTER III
FEMALE PLEASURE BY THE AID OF THE MAN,
BUT WITHOUT RECIPROCITY 151

CONCLUSION 165

INTRODUCTION

Charlie, twenty-eight years of age, brilliantly healthy, enjoying a moderate income, which he derived from the honest labour of his father in business, had as his mistress, Maud, over whose pretty head twenty-four summers had passed, She was the wife of a worthy fellow, whose icy temperament formed too great a contrast with that of his better half, so that it was no wonder that she should seek elsewhere that which she had no chance of finding in her husband's arms.

Charlie, free to do as he liked, was fond of the ladies, but in a tranquil fashion and brooking no delays, had met Maud at social gatherings, and she seems fitted for his simple, albeit lecherous, tastes. She, too, had remarked Charlie, who by his discreet, polite, and ardent manner, seemed well fitted to compensate her, without fear of scandal for the insufficiently of her husband, resulting from frigidity in the pleasures of love.

When two people are suited to each other, it is not long before they come to an arrangement, so a « liaison » was quickly established between the couple. Charlie possessed a neat little room, in a different neighbourhood from that of his residence, where could be found a bed, cosy arm-chairs, sofa, divan, chairs, cushions, rugs, and all furniture and necessary linen for the pursuits for which the nook was destined. All was arranged without useless luxury, but with care and cleanliness, and commodities of all kinds. Two little keys, of which Charlie and Maud each possessed one, allowed them to repair thither separately at the day and hour fixed by Maud, either by a sly « billet-doux » communicated at parties where the overs often met, or by a note that she carried herself to the little room, for it was understood that Charlie should go there every morning, between ten and eleven, except they had met overnight.

This state of things had lasted for eighteen months, the lovers having exhausted without lassitude every resource of free and happy passion. They agreed perfectly, in spite of time and satisfied enjoyment, absolutes and deserved. They had confidence in each other. Maud found that Charlie was not only a discreet and indefatigable lover, but also a man of firm mind, just and sensible, free of all prejudices, but respecting them for the sake of the worlds opinion.

Charlie recognised in Maud a good-hearted woman

not very capricious, but leaning towards the pleasures of passion in consequence of her fiery temperament, held in check, however, by a sensible brain; farseeing too, but desirous of learning. Their two souls were destined to agree.

One day, Charlie found in his boudoir a word from Maud, telling him that the same day she would come to pass the night, all the next and the following night, having obtained from her husband the permission to spend two or three days with a female friend a few miles out of London. She intented to go there on the third day and only stop twenty-four hours, so as to devote an entire day and two nights to love.

The two lovers had long desired to be able to sleep together at least one night and this had been impossible up to the present.

Charlie was delighted; it seemed to him as if he was now only for the first time about to really enjoy his mistress, although he had oftentimes passed many hours in bed in her arms, both of them in a state of nature, in the happy little lodging.

He awaited her coming therefore with impatient felicity, almost as if it was the first « rendez-vous » with Maud, who took care no to break her word, as she experienced in a like manner this tender feeling of her lover, so she arrived at seven o'clock in the evening.

Charlie had caused a light repast to be prepared, prettily laid out, but substantial withal. The table was near the bed; they gaily supped and retired between the sheets very early, so as to have more time for the amorous struggles, to which they gave themselves up with all the ardour of true, young, and vigorous lovers.

After having taken a large amount of voluptuous exercice, our two turtle-doves rested awhile and began to chat about the sweet pleasure they had had. They were both full of their subject. Curious little Maud began to speak first.

ENTRANCE TO THE TEMPLE

DIALOGUE I

ON THE PHYSICAL CONFORMATION OF MAN AND WOMAN

Maud. — You must confess, my dear boy, that you are a great libertine. I don't say that to reproach you, as, frankly, I get all the benefit, and not being a hypocrite I state the plain truth, but you seem imbued with the science of Venus to your fingers-ends, and I believe that there is not a single branch unknown to you.

Charlie. — I think you are right. I cannot help myself. From my most tender youth, it seemed to me that there were no other real pleasures than those given by the goddess of love, especially when a man had enough empire over himself no to abuse them. By this I mean that each one should know his own strength, otherwise definitive debility steps in, or premature old age, and impotency worse than death. I soon lost all scruples regarding the ways and means to arrive at enjoyment, and I tried to inculcate my ideas to all the women who succumbed to me, gently and warily, having due respect for their feelings of coyness and shame. I could never understand that one style of enjoyment should he more to he blamed than another, therefore I lent myself freely to all the capricious imaginations of my sweethearts. For they had various caprices, and all women who are loving and voluptuous and practice loves games have them too. In the same way, I persuaded them to give way to my salacious will, however extravagant the realisation of my dreams might he. Add to this that I had read everything, or nearly everything, that had ever been written in Latin, French, English or Italian on the art of voluptuous passion, and you are therefore correct in saying as you did, that there is very little, if there is anything at all, that I do not know in theory or in practice of this vast subject. The only thing that I have really never yet put into active experiment is sodomy, or any other kind of debauchery with my fellow men. I have always felt unconquerable repulsion for the carnal approach of a male, and that feeling has not yet left me. I wish all these who Lave masculine tastes plenty of fun and pleasure and blame them not because I believe that every desire is natural, that they become good and bad desires in merely a relative manner, and that each one should be free to amuse himself as he thinks best, as long as he does so without noise, scandal, or violence and harming no one. But for my own self, 1 do not understand the pleasures of man with man, while there is nothing which I am not ready to taste with any woman who pleases me.

Maud, — After what has passed between us, I can speak without circumlocution. You know that all women are full of curiosity? I am no exception to the rule. I should like — you will laugh at me perchance, but I care not — to be treated like an innocent girl desiring to learn all that you know so well of love and love's diversions, as if you were the professor of a maiden ignorant of everything, even of the difference of sex. My husband has taught me very little about all this scarcely a few words, so that it has happened that when out of doors I sometimes cannot understand certain words whispered in worldly conversation. I hear the sounds, without knowing their meaning. This vexes me. I look foolish, and no one likes to appear silly. When I talk of this to my husband, either I make mistakes, or he pretends I do, or what is more probable still, he knows very little more than me. Anyhow, he puts me off and there I am with my questions and no satisfactory answers. You are my first, my only lover; it is your duty to enlighten me.

Charlie « laughing ». — I willingly believe you, because you tell roc so, that I am at this present moment your only lover, but as for being the first...

Never mind, I am not your father confessor, I never trouble about the past life of a woman who pleases me, especially when her reputation is a good one. But that is not the question. You desire me to treat you like a perfectly innocent pupil, wishing to become learned in the science of Venus? Good, I can refuse naught that is in my power and that can be agreeable to you. But remember that first of all I must use technical terms without screen or veil, or double meanings, and I fear for your delicates ears.

Maud. — I know, sir, that, in the pleasures of science, the beginning is not all roses, but as I wish to learn, so as to be as wise as my master. I must perforce submit to walk at first mid thorns and briars. Fear not to wound my ears, any more than you have hitherto feared to wound other parts of my body, which it suited occasionnally to handle as you chose without thought of what I might suffer in consequence.

Charlie « laughing still ». — As you are blessed with such sweet resignation, fair lady, I will try all I can to satisfy you.

Therefore I begin :

THE SEXUAL PARTS OF MAN

Man and woman, though meant for each other, are constructed in a totally different manner, especially as regards the genital organs, which particularly distinguish one sex from the other and which are placed at the bottom of the belly between the thighs. These are called the « genitals », because they serve to engender the human race. The etymology is a Latin one and for that reason I need not tell it you.

The parts of the male are composed of a canal covered with flesh and muscles, forming by their mass a member which is more or less long and thick, springing from a kind of bag of skin containing two reservoirs shaped like beans, also more or less voluminous. This canal is called the urethra, and the entire organ is known as yard, prick, cock, viril member and a thousand other suggestive titles, such as : tiling, lance, dagger, spear, dart, perforator, pego, tool, John Thomas, piercer, etc. It grows out of the lower part of the belly, surmounting and between the man's thighs at a spot called the « pubis, » which becomes covered with hair at the age of puberty. It terminates with the nut or gland, which is a kind of acorn split at the exterior extremity, covered with a moveable skin that folds back at will, and during copulation, so as to leave this head naked and render the tickling of the sexual parts of the woman more enjoyable when it is introduced therein. This skin is fixed to the lower part of the nut, by a kind of membrane called the « fraenum » or fibre, which gets partly ruptured at the first venereal act of the man to permit the backward movements of this delicate covering, yelept prepuce, or « foreskin ». This fibre, which it shelters when at rest, is very tender, and to rub it or stretch it by pulling the foreskin strongly backwards gives the man great pleasure. The Beat of pleasure in the male is undoubtedly the sensitive top of his manly staff and by caressing and tickling it, you are sure at last to bring about the emission of his seed or spunk, by the orifice which is at the extremity of the gland. This seed is a whitish, viscous, salt liquid that, spirted by the virile member into the sexual parts of the woman, operates the miracle of generation and fecundates the female. By this aperture of the head of the gland the man also pisses.

The brown purse or hag is nothing more than a prolongation of the skin of the inner parts of the thighs, of that near the bum-hole and the cock, which also gets hairy at the age of puberty, and contains the reservoirs I just told you about. They are two glandular organs secreting the seed, spunk or sperm, made by the kidneys. This apparatus, the bag and its contents, in their entirety, are called the testicles, or the bollox, and there are other figurative names for it such as ball, etc., etc. Al ways on account of the two little round reservoirs. Beneath this bag is the continuation of the canal of the urethra, which extends from the neck of the bladder to the extremity of the penis, continuation, resembling a raised stitch, and on which is a sort of seam, is called the « perineum ». It divides the testicle bag into two parts and extends from the front edge of the arse-hole to the end of the prick. The whole length of the canal, or rather the flesh and muscles of which it is composed, swell up and stand out when the man has carnal desires, or when he feels the wish to discharge the superfluity of seed that he possesses. That is called « getting the horn » « getting stiff » having a « cock stand », or an « erection, » etc.

THE SEXUAL PARTS OF WOMAN

Woman's sexual parts are composed of a slit which is called the « vulva », from a Latin word signifying a door way, of which the two outer lips appear to be the folding doors. This opening begins at the bottom of the belly, where there is the « os pubis », or pubis bone, as in the male, and terminates at the perineum, near the hole in the bottom, or anus. This space comprises two large lips on the exterior of which, as well as on the pubis, is a growth of hair more or less abundant and of different shades, following generally the colour of the woman's tresses at the age of puberty, as with men in the same part of their bodies. Lifting open these large outer lips, we find within two little tongues, called small lips or nymphæ, on the summit of which, at the point where they meet, is a kind of little button or growth of flesh, resembling the top of the fibre of the head of a man's prick. It is called clitoris, button, etc., and is the seat of enjoyment for the woman, exactly as for the man the top of the prick and the fibre, which it resembles.

Beneath the clitoris, and close to the nymphæ, is a round hole with elastic ridges which forms a passage into the woman's body. This is the entrance of the vagina or neck of the womb, which is the name given to the interior parts of woman, where she conceives and where the child is nourished during gestation or pregnancy, generally lasting nine months. opening is partly stopped up when the woman is a virgin by a membrane called the hymen, unless they have broken it by pushing in a finger or any other rounded object.

Above the hole, under the clitoris, is another little aperture forming the opening of the canal which serves to void her urine. It is called « meatus urinarius » or female urinary organ. Between the external orifice of the vagina and the meeting of the large lips below, near the arse-hole, is a little sunken space called « fossa naviculeris ». The pair of small lips or nymphæ form above a triangular space called the vestibule. At the base of this triangle of which the clitoris forms the opposite angle and beneath it, the « meatus urinarius » is to be found. The point of junction of the big lips near the os pubis and the mount of Venus (name given to the little swelling formed by the flesh covering the os pubis) is called commissure of the vulva above. The junction of these same large lips beneath the « fossa navicularis » is called the fourchette or fork, or commissure of the vulva below.

The slit of the woman and all its organs together, as detailed above, is vulgarly called the « cunt ». It has, like the man's member, a number of facetious and figurative appellations such as sheath, furrow, in opposition to the cock, know as the spear, dagger, ploughshare. The cunt is also know as the cunny, pussy, cockle-shell, button-hole, etc.

Sometimes the name of the mount of Venus is also given to the same part found between the man's prick and the bottom of his belly.

We call seed, spunk, sperm, or seminal fluid, the liquid that is secreted by both men and women, which springs out of their reservoirs by the rubbing of their sexual parts together, and this discharge procures for both indescribable enjoyment. Some learned men pretend that woman has no real seed but only a moisture without prolific value. Besides these parts which form the female sex, women have usually on their breast two half globes which develop themselves about the age of puberty and become more or less large with age, filling with milk when the woman is a mother. These demi-globes vary in size and shape; they are sometimes close together, sometimes wide apart. Each of them is adorned in the middle by a pink button, whence issues milk which is given up to the eager sucking lips of the new-born babe. These buttons are called nipples and the globes are known as titties, teats, hubbies, dairies, bust, maternal hemispheres, breasts bosom, or « charms ». This last word applies to all the other beauties of the female form and sometimes to those of the male. Man is generally fascinated by the view of the feminine breast. He can scarcely ever view the naked titties, or even a small part of them, and still less kiss them, without feeling at once the desire to be carnally joined to the woman thus exposed, and he has an erection more or less strong according to his constitution. Carnal union takes place by the intromission of the manly prick in the feminine cunt. The action of the introduction and the movements made by both sexes, or by only one of them, to hasten the discharge or emisson of the seminal liquor, inevitable result and the desired end of this action, when continued long enough, is called fucking, poking, connection, getting up or into a woman, rogering, coition, copulation, having a go, etc. The buttocks of a woman also excite the imagination of the man immensely. They are generally worshipped and caressed just before fucking. These parts, very handsome when the female is well-built, with their rounded contours, their whiteness, and softness of the skin, are effectively often very attractive, and some men prefer them even to the cunt as an object of adoration.

For my part, I must tell you that I think woman is cunt all over and the contact of any part of her body pleases me, excites me and gives me desires, terminating by the act of enjoyment, which I willingly effect all over a woman, that is to say in or on any part of her person, so much do I love all and everything that is a part of this enchanting sex. On the other hand, my opinion is that a woman should have no repugnance in receiving all over her body the homage of the man to whom she consents to abandon herself. She should be unreserved with him, refuse him nothing and let him burn his incense on whichever of her altars that most excites his desire. He too, naturally, in grateful exchange of good will should renounce all individuality to the caprices of his mistress's imagination. This exchange should be complete and reciprocal.

Maud. — My dear friend, these are excellent principles and I frankly declare that they are mine, I think I have proved to you that indeed I do believe that there is no single part of my frame where you have not placed your lips, or caressed with your hands, and where you have not also, as you say, burnt incense to the god Cupid. All of my body, inside; and outside, where it is impossible for you to penetrate, has received the liquid and burning proofs of your lechery. You have not had my maidenhead in front, the bird had flown when you discovered the nest, but you have had the virginity of all the other parts of my body. As for me, I have felt you all over with my hands, caressed every bit of you with my lips and tongue and by the contact of my own entire self. My pussy has clung to you and rubbed against you in every direction, and so as my bosom and my bottom on every part of your person. You have readily lent yourself to all my whims and, I believe, I have satisfied all your lustful fancies.

Charlie. — Truly spoken, my angel. But I remarked that when talking of these things you seem to fear to use technical terms. That is ridiculous weakness between us two, assured as we are of being perfectly alone and safe from all surprise or spies. As we have no secrets for each other, why not call things by their proper names, which makes them more intelligible than, by wordly round-about phrases of pardonable use, perhaps necessary out of respect for conventionality? In society, it is quite essential to be more chaste in words than in action, but such conduct is useless in a « tête-à-tête » of lovers such as we are, when confiding abandon and loving frankness should reign supreme.

Say then innocently that my prick has touched upon every part of your person in every possible way, as your cunt, your hubbies, and your arse. Your hands have touched every bit of my body, and we have both emitted reciprocally in every part of ourselves that excited our desires of our caprices. Chastity of words is meaningless at the point we have both reached. If such is good and fitting in society, it is out of place and without motive during our meetings. I warn you therefore that you will be punished, if wishing, as you declare, to completely master the science of Venus, you do not start at once to speak the true language of the voluptuous goddess. In a word, you must call by their legitimate names the instruments used in love's temple and the true titles of all the rest. I shall slap your bottom as hard as I can and condemn you to caress and name three times, to get you used to it, any object that you do not in future call simply by its true designation.

Maud (laughing). — That will not be a very severe punishment, for you kiss more violently than you beat my bottom which you so cruelly threaten, but which you love too much to ill treat too greatly.

Nevertheless all you tell me seems right, but you must not be surprised that the habit of using very reserved language remains unwittingly, although it become useless or even ridiculous between us. Therefore, please excuse me and I will truthfully say that your cock, your hands, and your rake's mouth have touched every part of my body a thousand times; that you have inundated my cunt, my mouth, my hubbies, my hands, my arse, my buttocks, my thighs, my armpits, my feet, my back, my loins with your burning spunk; that I have received it spurting m my eyes, my hair, and my ears; that I have even swallowed some of it in many a moment of delicious delirium. That you yourself nave pumped and sucked my spermatic liquor with your mouth; that I have moistened your tongue, all your face, your hands and even your randy feet which have also frigged me. To sum up : that we have reciprocally covered each other with our mutual discharges. — And now are you happy? If you like, I will add that I take my solemn oath to the truth of this statement, and that I have experienced as much pleasure as you in all these wild bypaths of voluptuous passion, even to wishing often that you had a hundred pricks so that I might feel them simultaneously digging into me and ramming me all over, drowning me entirely with your seed both inside and out!

Charlie. — And I should like, my angel, to realise your desire, would it were possible for me to crush my whole being into your sweet body; in your velvet mouth; your pretty rosepink cunt; your delicious chocolate bum-hole and to caress all your frame with my hands and my burning tongue, while at the same time I would squirt therein countless jets of thick, rich seed which you would return with usurious interest as is your divine habit.

« Here occurs a pause in the dialogue. Our (dramatis personæ) worked up to fever heat, have suited the action to the word and have given themselves unreservedly up to the most delicious fucking. Our lovers exhaust themselves by repeated discharges in arse-hole, cunt, bubbies and mouth. They enjoy delicious [feeling], and countless tickling bouts on every part of their bodies, finishing up by a game of [Sixty-Nine] (No. 3, and Section, Dialogue V, page 134), during which

Charlie's staff disappears almost entirely in Maud's mouth, in whose throat he sends a last lightning discharge, eagerly swallowed to the very last drop in the excess of momentary lust, while Charlie sucks the divine essence of Maud till he wellnigh draws Mood, as the lecherous lover presses almost all his face into her cunt, carrying therein his stiffly held and lengthy tongue. At last, these two real lovers, overwhelmed by their delightful spendings, calm down a little, and refresh and restore themselves with some port wine and sandwiches; and then, languidly stretched out in repose, without strength to entwine their bodies, slumber peacefully, waking but four hours later, at about five in the morning, « After a yawn and a good stretch, the couple exchange kisses, but do not yet feel inclined to start on their merry games again. Besides, they wish to husband their ressources for the next night. Maud nestles her shapely head on Charlie's robust shoulder and begs him to continue his lecture. Willingly he consents, and Maud opens the debate, reminding her professor where he left off and telling him what impression he had made upon his pupil so far ».

DIALOGUE II

ON THE PLEASURES OF SOLITARY MASTURBATION SODOMY AND TRIBADISM

Maud, — All the details you gave me last night on the conformation of man and woman were for the most part quite new to me. Up to the present I had of course noted the difference of sex in my husband and myself without seeking to pry beneath the surface. My lord and master is far from being of a warm nature. He « does it » to me in a very slovenly sort of way. All he takes the trouble to do is to get between my thighs, put his prick, which is rather soft and thin, into my cunt, without having caressed it at all. He rides me and shakes himself up and down with only a shadow of lechery, spending with no thought of me, or wish to know whether I have done the same, so that often he leaves me in the lurch before I can « come », driving me mad with unsatisfied lust, hiring the sheets in sheer desire, and unheeding the state I am in, and which I try to calm by scratching with my finger-tips my poor little clitoris on the sly, while he snores by my side. He avoids carefully all talk of the pleasures of Venus, and to cut the story short fucks me as if he was taking a pinch of snuff, without any ardour, just as if he wanted to piss and no more. Fancy the difference I found when in your arms, when there is not a nerve in my whole body but what vibrates with pleasure. This difference has excited my curiosity and made me ask you for all this information. Continue to explain the theory of all these fascinating delights, which you know so well how to bring home to me by entrancing practice.

Charlie. — You must know, darling, that both man and woman, built as I have described, are born with the germ of the natural propensity to join carnally together. This germ is nothing more than the desire to get rid of the superabundance of seminal liquor that their loins have elaborated, and which develops more or less quickly when approaching the adult stage, according to their physical strength and the greater or lesser vigour of each and everyone, together with climatical influences and many other things too long to enumerate. In our temperate zone, it is generally about the age of fourteen that the boy or girl (a little earlier perhaps for the latter) begins to feel a new and unknow fire seething in their veins; the sexual parts begin to get covered with a hairy growth and this warm feeling means that the procreating liquid, just formed in the kidneys, is slowly reaching the genitals. The youth soon manifest the wish to approach the female, while she in her turn sighs for the presence of the male. If they have not been taught by more experienced people than themselves, they neither know the why or wherefore of these desires, but nature is at work and draws them together. If an opportunity offers itself, this same nature quickly teaches them to caress each other, at first in a perfectly innocent manner, and, then their brain being excited by the burning lava bursting to exude, they fuck, without knowing what they are doing: As the old proverb say: « Cock and cunt must come together ».

But if secret meetings are impossible, or if they have been instructed in the difference of sex by others, imagination goes to work, the spunk boils up more energetically and pushed on by these sensations without guessing the cause, their eyes and their hands are attracted to their private parts where the novel titillations have arisen. They provoke the emission of the seminal liquid by their sly touches which, at first involuntary, are continued by the force of the pleasure that is experienced. Now they freely renew the touchings and ticklings on their own bodies procuring such sweet and stealthy enjoyment, and so they become « masturbators ». Such is one of the names among many which are given to those who « frig » themselves, that is to say, who procure by the aid of the fingers, or in any other manner, but alone and without the help of another, the emission of the precious elixir. I say « in any other manner », as it may happen that a boy situated as I have stated, tossing about in his bed, agitated by the rising of the semen in his balls, or by reason of the dreams that the sap also generates, may rub himself against his mattress and by this friction sufficiently prolonged procure what is called a « pollution » : a complete discharge without the aid of the hands. In like manner, a girl moves excitedly about on her couch, until her bolster or any other object gets between her thighs. She may rub it against her swollen clitoris and move up and down until she loses consciousness in pouring forth her sweet essence. In both such cases, they begin again and again their pretty little games, which give a taste of the pleasures of paradise and finish up by finding the spot which, thus rubbed, is capable of, renewing for them the heavenly joys of emission. The hand wanders to standing prick or palpitating cunny and nature teaches them to do the rest. A callow youth fashions an imitation cunt with his fingers or anything else that is handy. The budding lass makes her finger do the office of a man's tool, or seizes a candle, an empty needle-case — heaven only knows what!

Maud. — Now tell me in as few words as possible what are the pleasures that each sex can thus procure all alone, or at any rate give me some slight idea of their secret manoeuvres.

MASCULINE SOLITARY MASTURBATION

Charlie. — By practice, I luckily know very little of the pleasures of masturbation, but I have heard its praises sung by school-fellows and will narrate to you all that was told to me by a poor devil who loved to frig himself so much, that he frigged himself to death. You know the ordinary fashion in which the prick is clutched in the right hand, lightly clasped, and the fingers go up and down, slowly at first, then the movement gets quicker, as pleasure begins to steal over the senses. The acorn is covered and uncovered in turn and the foreskin drawn down towards the root of the yard, so as to tighten the fibre, shaking lightly but speedily. The friction of the sensitive ruby top, and the strain upon the « fraenum », procure great pleasure, and when the discharge arrives, the jet spurts forth to a great distance giving double joy, by the titillation, which is excessive, and also by the sight of the furious fountain of manly essence.

To heighten the enjoyment, the left hand ought to travel beneath the bollox, pressing them lightly, shaking them, pulling the hairs, wandering along the « perineum », tickling the arse-hole and even pushing a finger therein, moistened with saliva. All these episodes spur on to fresh lascivious feelings and redouble the ecstasy, hastening the emission of the milky spunk and giving the highest degree of intensity to the final spasm of lubricity. Sometimes our frigging friend takes his rebellious prick with both hands and shakes it furiously upwards and downwards uncovering and covering the rubicund nut with prepuce until he discharges.

Another time he uncovers with one hand the head of his stuck-up comrade, pulling the foreskin towards the base. With a spittlemoistened finger of the other hand he gently rubs the tightened « fraenum » up and down, especially near the bead of the prick and all around the edge of the acorn. The supreme outburst is prompt and very agreeable by this method.

Another way is when he takes his cock near the top between his two outstretched palms, and moves then contrariwise, rolling his prick like the handle of a mop. The excitement produced by this exercise soon forces him to let loose his generative gravy.

And now also, reclining on his back, he forces his instrument back till it touches his belly and passes his hands up and down upon the prick, a cat's back, continuing until he spends.

Awhile he turns on his stomach, the prick pushed up captive between the belly and the bed. Up and down, and down and up he moves as if fucking. To add to the realism of the illusion, he takes his bolster, puts it beneath him as he would place a girl and keeps up the same dance as when his tool was 'twixt his belly and the mattress. Quickly thus, he reaches the desired gaol.

Again, lying on the bed face downwards, passes his cock between his thighs in the direction of his feet and, putting his hands behind him, moistens a finger of each hand, shoving one in his own brown hole while with the other he rubs the glistening head which he has uncapped. In this strange way, the prick being twisted, the viscous fluid flows slowly and with difficulty and the pleasure of the discharge lasts longer.

Another way — as the cookery books have it — to encompass the desired end. — The masturbator frigs himself standing up or seated, but passes the hand underneath his thigh to shake his weapon of which he can only grasp the head, drawing it towards him so that he spends behind himself. In all cases where the operator frigs himself with one hand, the other, should be used as much as possible to tickle the root of the prick, the balls, the perineum and the arse-hole, shoving in a finger if the chosen posture will allow of it.

Besides manual masturbation, known as onanism, from the sin of Onan and of which I have just given you a sufficiently exhaustive idea, he who has a taste for solitary and selfish pleasure, or who will have naught to do with womankind, either out of timidity, or by fears for his health or for any other reason, can employ other artificial aids to procure the happiness of the discharge. He can push his prick in a hole of a mattress, or a bolster, or any other soft stuffing; in muffs; in skins with or without fur; in short, or backsides, or any other orifices, nooks or crannies of statues and dummies, etc. A lump of meat, a hole in an orange; anything and anywhere where his imagination leads him will serve his purpose as long as he can spend by rubbing or pressing. Some triggers simply pop their prick between their thighs which they press together and shake until they are inundated with their own seed.

I think I have told you enough to enable you to fathom the resources of the masturbator, and to give you a slight idea of solitary joys of the male. We now will consider the female.

FEMININE SOLITARY MASTURBATION

She has no need to wet her fingers, either when rubbing her clitoris (which resembles, as I already mentioned, the top of the male organ, but is considerably more sensitive), or when pushing it into her cunt, for these parts are naturally always slightly damp. Indeed, the masturbating maid is soon ready. She whips up her petticoats or simply slips her hand through her pocket-hole, or any other mysterious slit in her gown, for I must not forget that the feminine dress-pocket changes its spots like the leopard, once in every decade, according to fashion decrees. Her slender third finger goes to work, lightly pressed on the magic button, and sometimes insinuating itself more or less in the cunny, where it is worked in and out, quickly or slowly, following the gradation of the pleasure she feels until she attains the venereal spasm and the delightful discharge, of which the proofs are rarely abundant. Some doctors have even doubted whether the female really ever emitted, pretending that what we take to be a gush of sperm is only a flow of liquid which does not emanate from the seminal canals but is only secreted by the prostatic glands, ressembling that which appears at the top of the man's prick when he gets an erection, serving to render the manipulation of the foreskin more easy, or if he has some weakness or inflammation. This colourless liquid is not the real seed and has no prolific virtue. Nevertheless, whether women have real spunk or only prostatic liquor, it is certain that, when they spend under the influence of any venereal act whatsoever, they have as much and more pleasure than their lords and masters, and as they lose less at a time, they can begin again more often and with much less fatigue. Thus it is that women are noted to be generally more able to resist reitcrated assaults extending over a short space of time.

Let me add that a man can only copulate when he has an erection. Without a cockstand how can his prick find shelter in a cunt; but woman is always ready to receive the peace-maker. She requires no preparatory erection, and as soon as she feels her stiff darling coming up the passage, his friction and her imagination does the rest. A woman can procure for herself the pleasure of the discharge, just as we can, by other means than manual ones. She has also the resource of the bolster and other similar objects which she can squeeze between her thighs, and rub her greedy furrow and her saucy clitoris against anything that comes in her way, from a brass knob or a bed-stead down to an odd finger of an old kid glove stuffed with wool. Some girls like to see themselves frigging and enjoy the solitary act seated, in front of a looking-glass. A leather or a camels hair brush produces enervating results and prolongs the salacious sensations. All is fish that comes to the female frigging net, as long as it ressembles in some slight degree the manly organ; any round wooden case, a carrot, a turnip, a saveloy, and Creole girls in tropical climes make a very tidy false cock out of a banana.

But enough on this head, or rather tail; I will lose no longer any time in discoursing upon what you understand, I am sure, perhaps better than I do myself?

Maud. — I think that you have draw a satisfactory picture of the pleasure that each sex can enjoy alone without the help either of the opposite species, or of his own, and that selfishly, as you truly stated. Now paint for me as well you can the image of the delights experienced by two persons of the same sexe : two males alone and then two women together.

SODOMY, OR MAN WITH MAN

Charlie. — I can only speak from hearsay of the joys of two or more men together, without women as I have never given way to this diversion, which never pleased me, although I have heard it praised by its votaries. Never has a masculine hand or any other part of a man's body touched any part of my naked frame, neither have I ever touched with my hand, or my prick, any masculine naked flesh. Everyone to his taste, so let me talk of those who feel differently to what I do.

Two men can frig themselves mutually in all sorts of ways they can rub themselves in all kinds of postures, one against the other, and thus obtain the emission of extract of manhood which, no matter how it is brought about, always causes more or less voluptuous sensations. But the most common fashion between these buggers, sodomites, catamites, bum-fuckers, pederasts — such are a few of the names bestowed upon those men who worship their own sex — is to abandon themselves to each other in turn, or sometimes each sticking to their original « rôle », by means of the prick of one of them in the arse-hole of the other. I say turn and turn about for those who like to be sometimes active and sometimes passive. The active one is he who sticks his cock up the bottom of the other. The passive victim receives the yard between his buttocks without flinching. And by « original role », I mean those who choose to be always either active or passive.

Such men take all those positions together, that present the arse to the attack of the others, either standing, seated or lying down. I shall give you a fuller description of these positions when telling you of dog fashion fucking between men and women, without laying stress on this topic which cannot interest you much, as I am certain you have no wish to hugger anybody, especially as you couldn't if you tried.

In all cases a man when buggering a comrade generally passes his hand in front of his victim, grasps his prick, frigs it, tickles his balls and the perineum, so that they both spend together, one of them in the other's arse, and the other in the palm of the perforating agent.

During all these libidinous acts the two men kiss each other, joining their tongues, feel each other's bodies in every part, lick each other all over, in fact treating each other mutually as if of a different sex. Sometimes one kisses the other's arse or, frigging him, he will push his fingers or his tongue in the arse-hole; they caress their balls mutually and the adjacent parts, nibble them, or the skin of the bag, sucking the little olives, etc. Another time they play at heads and tails, mutually sucking each other's cock, pressing it with their lips, and their teeth, and tickle the uncapped ruby head with the tip of the tongue, until a mutual explosion takes place in each other's mouth. At the same time their hands wander everywhere, exciting by all sorts of caresses and touches imaginable any part of the body within reach, reciprocally, but for preference always returning to the bollox, the root of the prick, and the neutral ground twixt purse and arse-hole, into which latter sepia-tinted retreat they madly dig one or more fingers. They fuck each other as well in the armpits and other parts imitating together as much as possible all that a man and woman can do as I will explain in due course.

Some of these gentry find great delight in forcing their victims to give them back in their hand, or even in their mouth, the spunk that they have just spurted in their backside. Some like to piss and even shit in the hand or even the mouth of another.

They often prefer to suck a prick when it has just left an arse-hole still reeking with whatever is lurking therein, and one of the pleasures of bottom-fucking is when the cock is found to have changed colour on leaving the tight hole, having become brown or yellow, from pink as it was on entering. There are many buggers who only care to get up a man just when he feels inclined to go to stool. They say in such a case that their cock finds a softer nook to wallow in and that the real pleasure of the true sodomitical arse-hole piercer is to plunge his instrument in a hot pudding obstructing the anus, bursting to force its way out. So before beginning their bottom-fuck they make sure by means of an investigating finger that the « egg » is there; that the rectum is full and the bird about to lay. In a word, these depraved fellows give themselves up together to everything that the most filthy and crapulous imagination can devise and the more horribly dirty it is, the more pleasure they experience. Some of these men, their brain weakened by such vile debauchery, prostitute animals to their unnatural lusts : dogs, cats, goats, cows, mares, etc. This is denominated bestiality. The depravity of these unsexed beings is unimaginable and you have no idea to what fearful extents their passions lead them.

They love to foregather and excite themselves in beastly emulation to invent fresh horrors. Three men will set to work at once. One is chosen to hugger a companion whom he frigs, while another will perforate the anus of the frigger. Then they say that he who is in the middle has double pleasure, because he is active and passive at the same time, receiving in his arse-hole the sperm of his friend, while he shoots his own roe into the bottom third accomplice, who at the moment of &e crisis inundates his hand simultaneously. A dozen or more form a ring sometimes, the backside of one turned towards the prick of another. At a given signal, each one effects an entrance into arse-hole in front of him, so that they all have a prick up their arse and their own cock is bottom. Thus they are all playing the dual part of master and slave. They feel and caress each other indulge in the most lascivious movements, join their lips and tongues as they turn their faces to each other, and the magic circle is only broken up when all have exhausted the reservoirs of nature to the last drop. This is sometimes called the holy chapelet of Corregio, from an obscene oil-painting attributed to this celebrated painter.

I must not leave this effeminate tribe vulgarly

know as « sods », which is a Cockney slang abbreviation for sodomites, without remarking that all those addicted to the Socratic vice are not quite so outrageous. Naturally enough, when we hear talk of buggers, the vision immediately arises of men violating the puckered, brown aperture of their fellows. But they are many pederastic amateurs who hold the culminating bum-fuck in horror. They love men like themselves, and give themselves up to men's lust simply for the sake of the prick. Yes, what they like is the standing prick; to suck it, to play with it, to show their own, to compare cocks and admire the tree of life in all its majestic beauty. They are worshippers of the Phallus. They adore the outward and visible sign of desire, and despise the hidden sources of love in the female, mainly because too much is really hidden away. Many such cock worshippers love women too. We may call them semi-sodomites. I just now remarked that Cockney slang shortens sodomite into « sod », but there is another sort of « argot » which is called rhyming slang, and it becomes doubly difficult for the profane when used in combination with ordinary slang. Thus a « sod » becomes a « Tommy Dodd » A prick is a « Hampton Wick » a cunt, a « Berkeley Hunt ». The venereal disease — the pox : « Jack-in-the-Box »; a

~ 51 ~

milder affliction : the clap — the « Horse and Trap ». arse is the « Bottle and Glass ». The Bollox : the « Tommy Rollocks, and so on « ad infinitum ». Not content with rhyming slang to slang, they shorten their jingle and the following sentence which I rapidly improvise will form a sufficient example for you. If you translate it properly to-morrow into the Queens English, you shall go to the top of the class or to the bottom of the bed, as you choose : « A Tommy took down his 'Round the Houses (Trousers), pulled up his 'Dicky Dirt (shirt) and showed his 'Bottle and Glass'. His pal got out his 'Hampton and shoved it up his 'North Pole' (arsehole) as it if were a 'Berkeley'. He catches hold his 'Rollocks' and says : « You know I've got the 'Horse and Trap' ». « Have you? » says the other, « well, I've got the Jack! ».

TRIBADISM, OR WOMEN WITH WOMEN

Do not think that women are less extraordinary in their pleasures among themselves without the help of the male. Those who fear the approach of a man, or prefer their own sex, are still more madly depraved than unsexed men. They put into play every resource of their frame and use foreign bodies too, to procure for themselves the happy dispatch, the sole desired end of male and females libertines. No stone is left unturned to obtain the spermatic result. They frig mutually, rubbing the clitoris with their fingers, which they introduce into each other's cunts, exchanging kisses, pressing bubbies, bottoms, and every, wart of the body, not forgetting to stick their digits up each other's little bum holes. They force into each others crack anything shaped like a prick. They get on top of each other, entwine their thighs and rub their cunts one on the other, pressing their hairy bushes till they are entangled together, clasped in each other's arms as if they are both of different sexes, and move and shake as hard as they can in convulsions of lubricity until they obtain the supreme happiness of the discharging crisis. Be it their liquid prolific quintessence, or simply prostatic, as some doctors says, the result is the same in the supreme moment of joy and they start off again until tired nature gives out. Ofttimes they wear a dildo, or godmiché, which is an ingenious little machine fashioned in the image of a man's cock, with hair and balls all complete, more or less artistically got-up and of different kinds of material, but sufficiently elastic, soft and smooth, and fastened by ribands or a strap to the lower part of the belly, exactly where the manly organ sticks out. The lady carrying the artificial weapon becomes the husband of a lecherous little bride, introducing, into her cunt this peculiar machine, which is a hollow tube of wood, tin or ivory, of a goodly size as thickness and length, and covered in leather or velvet. At the rounded top there is a little hole, the same as in the genuine article. The tube is filled with warm milk or any other syrupy liquid, and a piston, as in a syringe, serves to throw a jet into the vagina, at the psychological moment, when the woman whose parts are plugged up is about to discharge herself.

Nowadays these dildoes are made of india-rubber, with a ball-bag of the same. As this material is cold and Lard, it is generally left to soak before using in some hot soapy water. And then the balls are pressed and the instrument is filled with liquid. It now suffices to squeeze the balls at the proper moment to make the liquid spurt out by the hole in the accorn-top, absolutely like the true essence of virility. What gives great enjoyment to the woman in the use of this secret toy is that she can obtain a tremendous quickness of the movement to and fro, impossible with a man, however young or active he may be. But, of course, nothing equals the real thing, if it will only remain stiff and not collapse in the middle at the slightest pretext. A woman can strap the dildo on her heel and turning over on her back, dig away in her privates to her heart's content, and there is no act of parliament to prevent either sex being buggered with it. I have seen some very small one for little girls, or for teasing men's bum-holes and some of remarked size for special large Messalinas. Some are even arranged with a covering over the gland, imitating the foreskin. These are made for rich Jewesses, who out of curiosity want to try an uncircumcised pego without committing adultery. There exist also double ones, representing two pricks joined at the root and separated by a double set of balls, so that two women can each have an imitation prick in their cunt or arse-hole, as they choose, and so spend at the same moment as if they were hermaphrodites, male and female in one. If each girl presses the false testicles belonging to the india-rubber prick, each receives at once, or separately, the desired emission of the liquid they have put into the hollow canal. Imitation cunts have likewise been manufactured. They are made of india-rubber and are painted and bedecked with false hair exactly resembling a cunt. They can be pushed upon the prick with the hand, or the man can lie over them and simulate a genuine fuck.

Sodomites also use single and double dildoes in their orgies, either to take the place of exhausted pucks, or simply out of sheer lubricity, such as having them shoved up their backside while they are being sucked and frigged. Women often suck each other simultaneously, by lying over each other. One will be on her back, and, kneeling over her, the other will lick her cunt and press her own orifice down on to the lips of the woman she is sucking. The clitoris is tickled with the tongue, which is held out stiffly and made to quiver quickly on the sensitive button and all round the cunt and inside it, where they take as much of it as they can in the mouth and draw it up with an inward movement of aspiration, nose, the chin goes in too. They also tickle the arse-hole, and put in there their noses, tongues and fingers. They pinch each other, lick each other all over, and playfully nibble the cheeks of the arse and every other part that tempts them. Then again one will straddle over the other; either on her titties and ask to have her clitoris tickled with a rosy nipple, or else will sit or ride upon her mouth where the lips and tongue do their office as in the case of the « Sixty-nine » diversion I have just described, and during all this their hands are not idle; they travel everywhere, giving rise to voluptuous feelings by the sweetest titillations, varied and reiterated. There are no possible positions, or lascivious touches that they do not practise, every secret nook of their bodies is looked at, caressed, admired, kissed, pressed, pinched, sucked and nibbled. They try to become as one being and force their way into every opening of the body, exhausting their imagination to invent new methods of exhaustion of the body, by repeated discharges evoked by the most voluptuous and salacious games. These creatures treat each other as lover and mistress, or as husband and wife. Some prefer to play the masculine part and are always the « men » in this comedy of passion: others are ready for either sort of work, etc. They are called « tribades or anandrynes », from Greek words signifying a woman who is not for a man or who prefers her own sex. They are also known as Lesbians, gamahuching girls, and suckers, because they generally lick the genitals, a taste formerly supposed to be peculiar to the women of the island of Lesbos.

Some of these licking ladies do it out of sheer vice and devilry, others with mercenary motives. A poor Lesbian may sometimes get a rich woman into her power and force the latter to keep her in clover, either because the wealthy one is pleased to reward her for the pleasure found in sucking or being sucked, or else it is a case of blackmail. This passion is more flourishing than one might think, but it is very difficult to detect for obvious reasons. In all schools, workshops, convents, etc., there is more or less cunt-sucking going on, and governesses and servants often enjoy licking the virgin clefts of the girls left in their charge.

Now there are ladies who train canine pets and other domestic animals to lick their clitoris and their cunt until they spend. Others play with their dogs and monkeys, by frigging thein and frigging themselves, or by training them to fuck their adored mistress. Donkeys, I have been told, have even been used. The ass is strung up by the front legs by cords dangling from a ceiling or a beam. The lady slips underneath the suspended hoofs, either belly to belly, the back reclining on some convenient pile of sacks or bundle of hay; or else she goes on her hands and knees, her arse turned towards the donkey's gigantic fizzle which she frigs in either case and directs the monster prick into her greedy, gaping cunt, by the front, or in dog-fashion, but always holding it fast to prevent too much of it going in any farther than she can support without the danger of being split up. The ass then works bravely and she discharges several times while the donkey vigorously spurts his burning spunk, inundating her womb, bubbling up out cunt through its abundance, and trickling down her legs and thighs.

What more can I tell you of these strange doings? I can find no more to teach you. It is getting late. If you do not cafe to sleep a little before getting up, let us dress at once, have breakfast and go out and get a little fresh air. We can return this afternoon about three o'clock and then continue our studies again until we dine, between six and seven.

Maud. — Let us rise and have something to eat. I am quite ready and do not want to go to sleep.

(They leave the bed and, alter summary toilet enjoy a dainty breakfast. A hired brougham being in readiness, they go for a drive to Richmond, snugly hidden from prying eyes. While they are away, Charlie's discreet charwoman puts all in order and prepares the dinner ordered the day before by our hero. The lovers return at three p.m., and after Maud has taken off her dress, stays and boots and slipped on her « peignoir », and Charlie is at his ease in pyjamas, they recline on a comfortable sofa and resume the dialogue interrupted at breakfast time).

DIALOGUE III

ON THE VARIOUS WAYS OF VARYING THE PLEASURES OF LOVE BETWEEN MAN AND WOMAN

Maud. — The different and vivid pictures that you so graphically described this morning have enlightened me on many subjects completely new to me, as I am quite a novice with regard to all voluptuous pleasures except those that a lover can enjoy with a mistress who reciprocates his tender feelings. Those joys are the only ones that appeal strongly to me, so I must ask you to describe them fully and without restraint as they interest me more than anything else. You must, my dear boy, tell me all you know and explain every possible way that exists under the sun for an ardent woman and a vigorous lover to enjoy earn other fully, even if you have to recapitulate the different tricks that we have tried together. You understand, I want a complete lecture on this, to me, most important topic. Charlie. — It will take me some little time, my pet. Up to the present, in all the hooks I have read. I have never heard spoken of more than forty different ways. That is no niggardly figure, you must admit, but there are a lot more, although the conclusion is naturally always alike, while many resemble each other very much, at least to all appearances, but there are important differences when once put in action. Anyhow, I have promised to satisfy as fully as I can your curiosity and your wish for instruction. I shall therefore give you all details, sketching each method separately under a different and special name to help your memory and distinguish one from another. I confess that I speak from experience, as I have practised nearly all these delightful dodges myself, either because they pleased me, or in order, to satisfy the tastes of the various ladies with whom I have had loving connection. Between you and me, some of these sweet charmers were uncommonly lewd and naughty, and the frenzy of their lascivious brain was far from displeasing. So I begin without further preamble.

I shall divide this important subject into three chapters.

The first will treat of the different postures that two lovers, mutually helping each other, can put in action to procure complete reciprocal enjoyment. This chapter will be divided into two sections, of which the first is again subdivided into two paragraphs.

The second chapter will explain the various attitudes by which a man obtains the pleasurable discharge alone, by the caresses of a woman.

The third chapter will instruct you concerning everything relating to the diversity of means that allow a woman to obtain entire spending satisfaction by herself, but with the aid of the caresses of a man.

A general rule applies to these three important chapters, which is, that to fully appreciate the joys clung, the actors must be quiet and undisturbed, in a cosy, secret nook where there is no fear of surprise or prying eyes, and where they can find besides every possible commodity; a soft carpet; a good spring-bed, not too soft; divans, sofa, armchairs; ordinary chairs; footstools; cushions, and pillows. Plenty of water; two bidets; some perfumes; sponges; towels, and something nice and substantial to eat; wines, spirits and liqueurs.

Lastly, the principal thing to be done by the actors is to strip absolutely naked, both in a state of pure nature. Such is the only costume that is suitable for all true priests and priestesses of Venus.

CHAPTER I

POSTURES GIVING COMPLETE ENJOYMENT TO TWO LOVERS

SECTION I

POSTURES WITH INTRODUCTION

OF THE MEMBER

§ I

INTRODUCTION OF THE COCK IN THE CUNT

1 The Ordinary

Woman lies on her back, on a bed or anywhere else. She opens her outstretched legs and thighs, and receives between them her lover who at first kneels near the knees of his mistress, then he leans over, his legs and thighs united, upon her, supporting himself by one hand near the woman's shoulder. They are thus belly to belly, their faces close together. With the other hand the man gently opens the outer large lips of the cunt and direets between them his stiffly-standing prick introducing it just far enough to prevent it sliping out. He then withdraws the guiding hand, lets the upper part of his body fall on his mistress's breast, and hand lips glued to hers, supporting himself on one elbow, so as not to crush her by the weight of his body, his hands should wander all over her frame caressing every charm he can reach to, his tongue all the time working in and out of her mouth, meeting her velvet rosy tip as well. The active fucker now pushes up and down as sturdily as he can until the complete spending discharge of both the players, together if possible, but if not the woman first, and last of all the lord of the creation.

2 The Inseparables

This posture is almost the same as the preceding one, in theory, but when the woman is duly plugged she embraces the man by putting both arms round his neck (they were immobile and lying by her side in the foregoing) and crossing her legs and thighs over his loins, which was also omitted. This makes an immense difference in practice, especially for the degree of pleasure experienced, as the prick goes in much better in this second posture. The first one is generally used by cold couples and frigid fuckers, who do not like a woman to move during copulation, while the second is suitable for ardent combatants who, on the contrary, are only satisfied when the woman they are stroking answers every thrust with an upheaval of her arse and returns a hug for a squeeze, navel bumping against navel, until a mutual discharge ends the round.

3 The Ordinary with Legs Up

If the woman, instead of throwing her legs over the mans loins (as in the preceding attitude), will stick them straight up against his ribs, the feet pointing to the ceiling, forming thus by her legs and thighs two complete right angles with her body and that of her fucker placed one upon the other — as shown by a perpendicular line upon a horizontal one — the couple will demonstrate the « Ordinary, with Legs Up ». The rest as before, terminating with a double libation to the goddess of love.

4 The Baker

The woman lies across the bed, her bottom on the edge, with outstretched legs, one hanging outside and the other supported at the calf by one of the Lands of the man, who stands upright between beer thighs. With the other hand he directs his magic wand into the centre of delight, and then caresses the bubbies, the belly, the « mons veneris », and the clitoris of his lady fair, and any other beauties he may manage to reach, vigorously pushing his prick all the time in the little oven, until the loaves are baked and he has spent freely, while his partner shows her gratitude by spending with him.

5 The Saint-George

The man lies on his back on the bed and the woman straddles across him, on her knees. She covers with her cunt the uncapped prick of the male in erection, and gradually lowers herself upon it till their hairs mingle. Then she moves up and down, as if she was Saint-George himself on horseback galloping away to fight the dragon, The man seconds her in the furions dance by jerking his loins backwards and forwards, not forgetting to stroke with rakish hands every bit of her body. He feels her thighs, hips, her buttocks, and the lower part of the belly. He pats and presses every charm, until his caresses and their combined movements cause them to let fly a mutual gush of lovers balsam.

6 The Ordinary Reversed

The couple first place themselves as for « The Saint-George », and when the woman is fixed on the cock, she bends forward and stretches her legs out on those of the man, knee to knee. Her breasts press on the manly chest beneath her, and she encircles his neck or shoulders with her arms, according to her size. His arms in return are crossed over her back and he caresses as he chooses her loins and her buttocks. His fingers play about the crack of her arse and the little hole itself, which he should gently excite with a moistened digit. The result is inevitable, and the lovers die in each others arms, m the midst of a burning double inundation of fiery sperm. This is truly called the « Ordinary Reversed », as it is nothing more than the first position in contrary order : the woman above and the man below.

7 The Back-View

The man is on his back, the woman turns her back and rides over him, on her knees, near his. She settles down on his tool and mutually they dance up and down. Taking advantage of her position the woman plays with the man's balls, and he having both hands free can feel her back, loins and buttocks, of which latter charms he has a superb view, as the title of this pretty posture denotes. The lovers thus pleasantly occupied, and pushing properly, soon each of them furnishes an ample discharge, the proof of the pleasure they both experience.

8 The Stork

The woman stands upright, her bottom leaning against the edge of the bed. With her arms she embraces the man also standing in front of her, his lips on hers, breast to breast, and belly to belly. The man tucks one of her legs under his arm, presenting to her cunt his standing prick and guiding it with the hand that is free. Once inside that hand serves to clutch the woman's loins or her arse to support her and clasp her to him. Both now move in measure; their tongues meet and all terminates by a voluptuous spermatic outbreak on both sides.

9 The View of the Low-Countries

This resembles « The Back-View », (No. 7), Here the woman is riding the man in the same way, but instead of remaining straight up on her knees, she leans forward her face towards the man's feet, her bosom touching his knees and he therefore can see the entire arse stretched open, the hole of mystery, and the distended cunt, with his own prick moving in and out. He is quite at his ease to feel all these charms and tickle all round the genital laboratory, sharpening the work by prodding a finger in the anus that seems to him to be the eye of a Cyclops staring him out of countenance. To reward him for his caresses the lady tickles his bare feet with her velvet tongue. Now you know what is meant by « The View of the Low-Countries », and this enchanting prospect, combined with the couple's cunning caresses, leads the fuckers on to furious movements, of which a copious and mutual discharge promptly becomes a natural consequence.

10 Speared Sideways

The man is seated on the edge of a chair, his legs slightly open : prick stiff and ready. The woman stands sideways, her right leg between those of the man and the other crossed over his left thigh. She holds her left arm round his neck from behind and the man takes her hand with his left also. With the right, she guides into her nest the staff which has presented itself between the top of her thighs from behind. She stoops a little when the junction is complete and can then frig herself with the right hand, or caress the face of her lover, who with « his » right can play with her loins and her arse, as she is partly seated on her lover's right thigh. This play and the reciprocal movement soon bring about the mutual sweet emission of the amorous liquor.

11 A Woman's Prayer

The woman kneels on the edge of a low bed or sofa, the thighs well apart. The man stands in front of her, holding his stiff prick which he directs into the happy opening. With the other hand he holds her round the back, above or below the shoulders according to his height, and bringing it round to her breast, he plays with the nipple if he can, while the woman also embraces him with one arm or both. They are thus face to face, their tongues entwined, and the man can caress his sweetheart as he likes, back and front, with the hand that served to guide his priapus. During this time their arse and loin movements prove that they are far from idle, and a prompt, mutual and, delicious ejaculation gives irrefutable proof that the prayer of the woman has been heard.

12 A Man's Prayer

The man takes the place of the woman in the preceding posture : on his knees, leaning slightly backwards, his buttocks touching his heels on the bed or sofa, where the woman mounts facing him. She opens her thighs, approaches her belly close to the chest of her valiant fucker, encircling his neck with her arms, and he puts his bands under the cheeks of her arse, supporting her. He opens the lips of the cunt from underneath, into which he directs his erect instrument. Then the woman bends forward to aid the complete introduction and the man thus has before his mouth his mistress's heaving globes, against which he can press his face. He lifts up with his hands and lets fall again her arse, which he is holding, so as to let his prick go in and out of its agreeable sheath, but never slipping out entirely. The lovers at last combine their movements and in a few minutes they feel their veins let loose floods of that liquid, which causes such pleasure when it escapes and which was what the man was praying for in his turn.

13 A Woman's Resignation

The woman lies on her back, her arms crossed below the breasts, the loins on the edge of the bed, the legs and the bottom free. The man stands up between the woman's legs, tucking one under each arm. He opens the cunt-lips, plants his prick therein and pushes forward without the woman making the least movement When he is well in the citadel, his hands and fore-arms are at liberty to excite by all kinds of sly touches the arse and the rest of the beautiful, indolent resigned charmer. She cannot resist this play very long and soon her discharge mingles with, that which her lover bedews her secret charm's, rendered full of lewd feelings by this sweet unction.

14 The Elastic Cunt

The woman sits on the edge of the bed. Leaning backwards a little, resting on her hands. The man stands between her thighs, lifts her legs off the ground, takes one of her feet in each hand and holds them straight so that her heels touch her own buttocks. In this position he puts his prick in her cunt and while he shoves backwards and forwards, he lifts up, kisses, holds, aparts and brings together alternately the feet he holds, one after the other, or with a contrary movement, or both together. This creates delicious movement inside the cunt, rendering also the friction of the tool much more delightful, making up for the deprivation of all the other habitual caresses from which the lovers are momentarily debarred, their hands being occupied and their faces far from each other. But the exciting filiations are doubly exquisite inside the temple of love, on the altar where the sacrifice is made, and the libation soon flows from the spermatic canals of the two worshippers.

15 Winnowing on the Belly

The woman lies on her belly, crossways on the bed, legs and thighs outside and well apart The man stands up between her legs, which he clasps and lifts to his hips. He holds them with both hands near the knees; they stick out horizontally behind him. From underneath, he directs his cock in the beauty's bulls-eye, and pushes up and down as if he was winnowing. He can see his charmer's back, and she can turn her face towards him; his eyes feast on her delicious arse which, at each sturdy stroke of his loins, jumps up like a winnowing fan or basket and wit wriggling movements, the sight of which would make an eunuch spend. So the work goes on, winnower making such lusty efforts that he soon terminates his task, and instead of the dust that winnowing usually produces, he squirts into the entrails of the woman the divine dew of love and she pays him back with interest.

16 Winnowing on the Back

This is the same posture as the foregoing, but reversed. The woman lies on her back instead of being on her belly and the man does the same as before. He holds her legs by the calves and is face to face with her. Instead of having the view of her back, loins and arse, he can gloat over her breasts, her belly and her mount of Venus. In this encounter the woman herself guides the prick within her secret retreat which is always very acceptable to a lover. The rest as before, arriving quickly at a similar result — a reciprocal and voluptuous discharge.

17 The Wheelbarrow

The woman lying down, throws her hands forward, either resting them on a footstool mounted on castors, or better still on the middle of a snort stick hearing a wheel to left and right The man stands behind her, fucking her dog-fashion, that is to say: opening the cheeks of her arse he gets into her cunt from underneath the arsis hole. (See further on : « Simple Dog-Fashion »). Then he clasps her legs and tucks them under his arms leaning on his hips. He pushes in front of him, forcing his prick into the womans cunt and she, supported only by the stool on castors, or the stick and the wheels, rolls forward exactly like a wheelbarrow. The man can conduct her where he likes, fucking her as he goes, enjoying the perspective of her back, loins arse and the seat of their mutual passion, lithe woman is strong enough to support herself, with one hand only, she can either frig herself with the other or gently agitate from underneath her lover's balls, to bring on his discharge quickly, as the position for her is rather fatiguing and she evidently desires to reach the end of her tether as soon as possible and wind up by a welcome inundation.

18 The Wheelbarrow Reversed

This posture, although a little less fatiguine for the female, is hardly ever put in practice. This remark applies to a few otters, although I shall describe them all. The reason is because the prick does not get far enough in the cunt being only suitable when the man's cock being too long, the woman tries to engulph but a small portion by positions that keeps the man a little way off. But alas! Say the ladies, this too great length of the member is so very rare, that we can only speak of it from hearsay. Anyhow, this is how this position is arranged : the woman lies on her back on the carpet, resting her head and shoulders on the stool with castors. She passes her hands behind her head and seizes the outer edge of the stool. The man stands between her open thighs, his face towards her. He lifts her up by the calves and with his arms clasps her legs against his hips, directing his prick in the cunt that the woman presents to him in good order, as she offers her arse and stiffens her loins. The rest of the pleasure is the same as for the simple « Wheelbarrow » posture I have just noted. This one is called the « Wheelbarrow Reversed » to distinguish from the original.

19 The Trot

This posture resembles « The Saint-George » (No. 5). The man, instead of lying down, is seated on the edge of a sofa, leaning backwards, his head and shoulders supported by cushions. The woman is not on her knees. She mounts upon the sofa, her face to his, squatting down over her partner, whose shoulders she holds. He passes his hands under the lady's arse, very much as in the posture: « A Man's Prayer ». (No. 12), and supporting her thus, he directs at the same time his prick in the warm shelter. She moves up and down with a lilting and dropping movement of the body, but careful not to let Her prisoner escape, imitating the movement of a man on horseback gaily trotting, which gives the title to his very amusing posture and does not fail to produce a superb mutual ejaculation of burning sperm, which wets the root of the prick and the balls as it runs down, because the cunt is too much open by this position. So the greedy cavity regretfully lets all escape.

20 Empalement Backwards

This is the foregoing posture reversed. It resembles a « Back View », (No. 7), without being exactly the same. In No. 7, the woman is on her knees. Here she is on her feet, crouching over the man's prick, her back towards him, so that the cunt is forced out in a much more satisfactory manner. Her legs and thighs are forced up left and right of her belly instead of dropping down as when she was on her knees on the bed. The lovers gain at least an inch of prick. The man need not fear that his fuck-stress will fall backwards, and if she did, she would fall upon him and not hurt herself. He supports her with one hand and the other serves to press and feel all her charms within his reach, in front or behind. She can enjoy the backward and foreward movement of the prick and can frig herself and even play with the root of the cock, and the balls of her lover. This posture is a delicious example and procures extraordinary delights for the actors by the reciprocal discharges it cannot fail to bring about.

21 Empalement in front

This posture is very much like « The Trot », (No. 19). Here the man, instead of being seated, is lying down and the woman rides across him crouching down, her feet on the bed, her face turned towards that of the man. Instead of holding on to his shoulders, she clasps one of his hands. Thus they have each one hand free, and they can indulge in mutual caresses. She, turning a little to one side, can seize the root of the man's prick and his balls by passing her hand underneath her thighs. He can enjoy all the charms of the front of her body : her breasts, thighs, belly, and her mossy cleft, without hindering their natural fucking movements. On the contrary, they quickly lose their strength and their essence at this sweet game, in the midst of the most intense and delightful sensations.

22 The Roman Chair

The man is seated on a low chair. He leans backwards, each hand supported by another chair behind him: the legs are outstretched and he has a stool at the side of his feet joined together. The woman straddles across his thighs, her face turned towards his. She guides his weapon into her cunt and when he is well in, she also leans backwards, stretching out her legs and resting her feet on the rail of the chairs that serve to support her lovers hands, while she places her hands behind her on the chairs that stand on either side of his feet. Their two bodies are crossed, leaning backwards, the legs stretched out contrariwise, but the lovers are joined by the prick and form a figure resembling a Roman Chair in the form of the letter X, giving the name to his eccentric posture which, like the others, quickly forces the reciprocal ejaculation and its accompanying transports.

23 The Herculean Feat

The man stands up, his cock ready, so stiff that it looks if it was trying to fuck the navel above it. The woman, undismayed, is in front of her lover, impatient with desire. She throws her arms round his neck, bends down and then springs up, legs and thighs wide open, throwing them round his body near the hips, joining them behind his loins, her heels on his arse with one hand, guiding his tool with the other and plunging it within her, till their hairs are mingled together. He then presses her towards him by the cheeks of her arse, and supports her loins to keep her fixed to his clutch. Thus upstanding, he swives her manfully and she returns each shove of his arse till the abundant double libation is poured out, proving the battle to be a drawn one. It can be well understood why this posture is called « The Herculean Feat », as there are few men sufficiently adroit and athletic to put it in action with a stoutly built female.

24 The Crossed Scissors

The woman lies on her side, half across the bed, her elbows leaning thereon on the same side, crossing her fore-arms on the pillows. The man, standing near her feet, takes her right leg in his left hand, lifting it off the bed and passing between the bed and this same right thigh of hers, which comes thus against his belly. His right hand is directed beneath her loins between her and the bed, lifting her a little and causing her right thigh to fall outside the bed and it is drawn away from the other which he supports. The right leg naturally passes between his calves. Then, with the left hand, which just now supported her left thigh, he directs the arrow to the target, and by force of the position he fucks her sideways in dog-fashion. Once therein he treats her like a hungry lover. The lady turns a laughing, provoking visage towards him. She is hugely excited by this position which leaves her well-nigh powerless to assist him, but nevertheless the merit of the conclusion is proved to them by a copious emission. The title of this posture comes from the crossing of the lovers' legs, resembling two pairs of Scissors, the blades opened and crossed.

25 The Sharpshooter

When executed this posture is akin to the preceding one if reversed a little on the man from left to right, The man lies outstretched upon the bed, the right knee uplifted. The woman mounts over him, crossways. She puts her right knee on the bed, passing her folded leg underneath his lifted knee, her foot towards the other edge of the bed. By this manoeuvre her cunt is just above the prick half dog-fashion. He passes his left hand under her thighs, guides his member into the proper place, lifts up her loins to force his way, and pushes up and down, feeling her beautiful arse with the right, tickling the arse-hole a little, while his left can be busy with her hubbies and the disengaged parts of her cunt, She supports herself with the right hand behind the uplifted knee of her lover, stroking his face with her left. All soon terminates as usual, with a double volley. It is the position of the knee of the woman on the bed that causes the appellation : « The Sharpshooter recalling the command : « Front row. Kneeling! » Recommended to military men.

26 Lazy Style

The woman lies up on the bed, her arms crossed over her head on the top of the pillow, her arse and loins are turned away from the side where her lover reclines, crossways, but his face towards his mistress. He gets between her thighs, lifting one up and passing it over his hip. He brings his prick to the mark, by passing his body above the thigh of the woman. So lazy that she does not move. He then places one arm on her shoulders and with the other strokes her bosom, neck and face, and gives her a fair rousting, which obliges her to finish by discharging, as she feels her lover inundate her with burning essence of manhood, an excellent medicine to cure laziness in the female.

27 Lazy Style Reversed or in Dog-Fashion

This is the exact opposite of the foregoing, i.e. it is now done dog-fashion. The woman lies half across the bed, turning her back, head and shoulders on the pillow which is placed rather high up. The man appears at her feet, drops on the ground her leg which is nearest to the edge of the bed, seizing to the other at the knee and, passing behind, places it on his hip, the point of the loot resting on a convenient stool. He passes one arm under her shoulders, and she has her arms nonchalantly thrown to the right and to the left. Passing his other hand in front he guides the peacemaker under shelter, introducing it from back to front, and afterwards this same hand caresses her bubbies or the environs of the grotto and the clitoris. He kisses her mouth, her half-shut eyes, and all her face. She lets him work his sweet will without making the least movement but in spite of this immobility all ends by her discharge, showing her pleasure by the thrill of her arse and the nipping of her cunt sucking up the spunk which bursts from her fucker's ruby nozzle.

28 Double Lazy Style

The woman lies on her side, passing her arms round the neck of the man who lies on his side too, facing her. He passes his legs and thighs between those of his companion, clasping her round the body under the arms, after having, of course, introduced his stiff visitor into the nook of joy, which opens all alone by the way the male has installed, himself between her ivory columns. The actors go to work mutually but without undue bustle or hurry, joining their mouths greedily, but soon are warmed up by the soft reciprocal heat of the magnetic attraction that draws the sexes together. After having tasted a few moments the happiness of feeling their frames thus joined together without any painful effort, their movements quicken in spite of themselves and the torrent that rushes from both sources obliges them to embrace with a fury which is quite a contrast of the indolent commencement of the struggle.

29 Double Lazy Style Reversed

This is the same system as in the preceding directions, but the woman, lying on her side, turns her back to her lover who, also on his side and with his belly to her arse, lifts up her thigh — the one that does not rest on the bed — and places himself between the sturdy pillars thus separated, advancing his legs and knees forward beyond the woman's body in front of her. Her uplifted thigh now rests upon her lover's hip; her bottom is in front of his prick, which he directs dog-fashion from behind into her cunt, plunging it to the hilt and now fucks grandly in this commodious and far from tiring position. His hands are at liberty to press and pat ail the surrounding beauties, especially the redundant cheeks of her arse which rub against his pubis and which he can caress and slap at will. His partner soon feels the effect produced and experiences herself the discharging delights, when the neck of her womb palpitates and is sprinkled by her lover's elixir.

30 The Game of Touch

The man sits on the bed or on the ground, his back and loins supported by pillows or cushions, his legs apart, and his dagger, like a Freemason's, threatening the sky. The woman squats between his thighs, stradling her white pillars over the brawny limbs of the man. She crams his tit-bit into her orifice, leaning against him. The two lovers entwine their arms and advance their lips to fence with their tongues; the woman leaning her arms on her champions's shoulders. With the aid of her frisky back-side, she makes the backward and forward movements in the style of those made by children as a preliminary to their games of « hide and seek » or touch », when it is necessary to find out who is to go and hide or to run and try and place a hand on one of the other players. The man is not ungrateful and returns blow for blow, so that this simultaneous action soon starts the couple's pumps to put out the fire that devours them, making it impossible for them to decide who « touched last ».

31 Contemplation

A variation of the last posture. The woman, seated as before said upon the man, throws herself backwards and leans her head and her shoulders, which are lifted a little, upon a cushion placed between her lover's feet. He also leans back, but only a trifle. The woman stretches her legs entirely out in front of her on her lover's body, placing her heels upon his shoulders. He clasps her legs and opens or shuts them just as he feels inclined, either to inspect the work going on, or to close his prick in her vice-like pussy. Hence the title : « Contemplation ». Leaning on their elbows, they both shove their bottoms forward and backward, enjoying the sight of the junction, but soon their eyesight becomes dimmed, they can hardly see; their pupils turn up towards heaven, their bodies stiffen, and our lovers remain motionless, after having let fly a flood of amorous liquor, in the midst of the wildest, sweetest joy.

32 Dog-Fashion Sideways

The woman lies full length of her side, on the edge of the bed horizontally, her bottom outside, the legs and thighs folded half perpendicularly to the couch, so as to give full prominence to the arse. The man stands upright behind the tempting buttocks, lifting the uppermost thigh, by seizing her foot by the heel and dragging it backwards. The other hand is passed in front to direct his prick from behind into the cunt, and when placed therein, he is at liberty to pinch and stroke all the rosy flesh within his reach. He frigs the reclining beauty and she holds his head with one hand, her other arm being on the pillow. He feels her belly, her hubbies, her backside, her loins, etc., at the same time driving home his piston. Its vigorous in and out action produces the usual effect, bringing into play the double fountains of burning spunk, with their attendant ecstacies.

33 Dog-Fashion Kneeling

The woman is « all fours », upon her knees and elbows, on the bed or on the floor. The man kneels behind, adjusting his prick between the lips of his charmer's cunt, which he opens. He can see toe rosy retreat well, because her head is lower than her arse. When installed, he can, by putting a hand in front, frig the button of the cunt while he fucks, and tickle her hairy mount, while with the other hand, by leaning forward a little over her back, he is able to take hold of her globes, and tickle the strawberry nipples, kissing and licking her shoulders and spine. The woman, not to be behindhand, can support herself on one elbow only, and pass the free hand between her thighs to gently daddle the balls belonging to the prick within her. She must lean forward also just a little more, as the more the woman is bent double, the more the entrance of her cunt is facilitated, enabling the lovers to gain one or two inches more of length of prick, especially if her fair forehead entirely touches the floor or mattress. By this position it must not be forgotten that not one drop of the divine elixir of their reciprocal gush is lost; all remains in the thirsty cunt, to their great and mutual delight.

34 Ordinary Dog-Fashion on the Bed or Standing

This is a variation of the preceding way the woman, instead of being on her knees, is flat on her belly on the edge of the bed, legs, thighs and arse outside; her feet resting on two small stools or hassocks, forming « Ordinary Dog-Fashion on the Bed ». Or she may be standing, leaning forward, her hands resting on some handy object that forces her head to be lower than her bottom; thus showing us « Ordinary Dog-Fashion Standing ». In both these cases, the man is always behind the woman's arse, ready to introduce his prick from below the brown hole into the cunt, of which he tenderly operates afterwards as I stated in the last attitude.

35 Dog-Fashion Straight

Now the man kneels and the woman approaches him backwards, presenting her backside to his face. She opens her legs and thighs, passing her hand between them to seize his swollen prick, which she directs herself, introducing it into her cunt from back to front Then the man clutches her hips and helps to claw her on to his cock She pushes quickly forward and backward, up and down, and leaning in front passes her hand between her thighs to play with the stones and the lower end of the reeking dagger. Soon both overflow voluptuously. This posture is so called, because the woman is nearly upright.

36 The Spikey Chair

The man sits on a chair, almost on the edge. The woman turns her hack to him and comes and sits down on his lap, but she bends forward a little at first, to allow her workman to adjust his tool in her cunt from behind her arse to the front When it is quite sucked in, the woman lets herself fall back seated on his thighs, turning her face towards him so as to suck his lips and tongue. You now see why posture is dubbed : « The Spikey Chair ». The man's hands at liberty serve to feel all the lady's charms. He can press her breasts, tickle her nipples, caress her lithe body and exciting her and himself by these lewd touches, added to the joint action of their loins, they are soon forced to open their sluices together with voluptuous abundance.

37 Dog-Fashion Flying

The same as in this preceding description, with the exception that the woman, instead of remaining with her thighs upon those of the man, opens them as wide as she can and throws her legs behind her right and left of the chair upon which he is seated. The man passes one arm round her body to prevent her from falling forward, as the posture forces her to do. The remainder as before, but the prick enters better and both the lovers profit thereby. As the woman leans the upperpart of her frame forward and her legs are stretched behind her feet off the ground, only supported by the man's arm that clasps her to his middle, she may be said to be almost flying.

38 Dog-Fashion Upright

This posture is the same as « Ordinary Dog-Fashion Standing », (No. 34), but here the woman, instead of leaning forward, draws herself up as soon as she feels her cunt properly plugged and turns her face towards the man, giving him her tongue, while the hands at liberty caress all they can but above all the breasts. To fully succed this position the male should be blessed with a very long perforator, otherwise he will find himself outside at the least movement; the actors being both on their feet. The prick, to rest properly in the cunt, must be bent, and the warm nook is a good distance away from the male, through the female's arse pressing against his belly and pubis. Such is a fine style of coition for those rare individuals who possess too long a penis, and obviates the use of the soft rings they are forced in ordinary copulation to put round the lower part, to prevent too much going in and bursting the womb. But with the usual size cock, any woman who may feel during the posture of upright dog-fashion or standing, that the peacemaker is escaping, must hasten to lean forward to put him back in prison, forming thus once more the « Ordinary Fashion Standing », (No. 34).

39 The Cock-Horse

The man sits on the edge of a chair, the shoulders leaning on the back of it, the knees well forward. The woman straddles across him, her face to his, and lowers her cunt on his stiff rod until it disappears within. Her legs are passed behind the chair and she throws her arms round his neck, so that her heaving semi-globes are close to his face. His hands, after they have helped to introduce the prick to its natural shelter, eagerly pet, slap, stroke and pinch all the beauties of his rider that he can get at, and he must not forget to introduce a frolicsome digit into her palpitating bum-hole. To reward him, the woman, by lowering her head, can plunge her warm tongue between his teeth. Now the pace gets furious, she « rides her cock-horse to Banbury Cross », and so gives the name to this fascinating combination, and they soon reach their destination, each marking the end of the journey by a discharge from the venereal reservoirs.

40 Nailed Woman

The lovers take up the same positions as in the preceding encounter. When all is ready and John Thomas it at home, the man lifts up the woman's thighs, an arm under each knee, supporting her by the hands, grasping the rotundities of her posteriors and pushing them up and down. She, clasping his neck, kisses him, tips him the velvet, and sucks his lips until the spunk flows from both and gives them complete voluptuous satisfaction. The title of this posture comes from the fact that the woman seems as if she was immovably fixed to her lover, or « nailed » to him.

41 The Bastard Cock-Horse

Is so called because this posture is made up of the elements of several others without completely resembling anyone exactly. The man sits in the same way as for. « The Cock-Horse ». (No. 39), but on the middle of a low sofa, leaning back a little on some cushions. The woman gets across him, kneeling as in « The Saint-George », (No. 5), but not straddling down over him, for that would be « The Trot ». (No. 19). But remark that here the man is seated and not lying down, as in No. 5. Their bodies form a right angle of 45 degrees separating their two faces. The present posture resembles more that of. « The Ordinary Reversed », (No. 6), the only difference being that in the latter the legs of the lady are stretched out and the lovers are lying at full length, while here the man is seated and the woman's knees are bent.

42 The Cock-Horse Crossed Straight

Can only be performed with a form or narrow bench, up on which the man lies on his back, at full length. The woman rides across his middle, her legs dangling on either side and her face turned towards that of her lover. His hands, unoccupied rummage all the treasures in view, but principally the secret one where the woman has popped in his cock herself, being commodiously placed to do so without his help. He then throws up his belly, like a fish out of water, up and down, and she gently wriggles her backside backwards, and sideways, and round and round. These movements, if well-timed and in measure, are delicious, and procure such extraordinary sensations that the couple quickly give each other reciprocal liquid proofs of melting delight.

43 The Cock-Horse Crossed Reversed

Absolutely the same as in the preceding sketch, only the woman's face is turned towards her lover's feet. This variation enables her to put her hand between her thighs and take hold of his balls and root of the prick, with one hand, or with the two. The man, deprived of a view of the baby manufactory, and the breasts, can feast his eyes on her back, loins, and buttocks. They both move as in the foregoing attitude and obtain the same result : a mutual delirious discharge, and just as agreeable.

44 < T > Upside Down

The man sits on the bed, his legs stretched out straight. The woman rides upon him, her breast to his, mouth to mouth. She passes one leg to the right and one to the left of the man's, straight out behind him. Their two bodies cemented together, their leg's pushed forward as far as they can go, the woman's behind the man, the man's behind the woman, gives to the view of the couple in profile the form of a capital T upside down ($\perp$) thus baptising this posture. Their hands are free to place the cock where it should be and the picture once realised, they can mutually caress, and suck each other's breath, work their loins and bottoms and meet inevitably at the desired goal with a charming spermatic give-and-take.

45 Sideways

The man is placed on the edge of an arm-chair across it; his back reclining against one of the arms. The woman sits also crossways, one arse-cheek on the man's knee, holding on to his shoulder. Her other posterior with uplifted thigh reposes on his belly, her foot on the arm of the chair to enable him to introduce his prick in her cunt from underneath. She leans her other hand on the back of a chair behind her, on the bottom rail of which her lover places his feet to support her. With one hand he clutches her by the lower part of her back and with the other strokes, feels and pats her breasts, belly and even round her hairy gap, although his prick is fast held within it. The lovers are hard at work and, as ever, with gasps and sighs of rapture, finish by discharging admirably.

46 The Good Wife and Mother

This posture is almost a copy of the preceding one. The woman is half-lying across the bed, leaning on one elbow; the child she is suckling is fixed to the opposite breast with greedy lips; pillows support her head and shoulders; her legs and thighs are outside the bed. Her husband comes to her side, lifting up one of her legs which he places on his shoulder and the other rests on his knee. By this tactic he fucks her dog-fashion, sideways. His legitimate or illegitimate spouse gives way to him with pleased obedience, still suckling the infant, who is agreeably rocked in his mother's arms by the thrusts of the man and the regular upheaval of the maternal arse. The woman gives down her sperm at the same time as her milk, softly begging the father of the babe whose prick is throbbing, ready to let loose, not to discharge in her vibrating cunt, but to empty the barrel of his gun outside, so as not to break the child's feeding-bottle, by getting her again in the family way too soon, impoverishing her milk.

47 Pedestal Fucking

On a pedestal, or a fragment of a column, a cushion is placed; the corner of a table will do as well, or any other piece of furniture about two feet and a half high. The woman sits on the cushion; the man is before her, between her thighs which she lifts, so that her knees come up to his armpits. She holds him round the neck, crossing her legs behind his back and he, standing up, directs his prick in the willing cunt, which, distended to the utmost, awaits it impatiently. He then clasps her to him with both hands by her backside and loins. The woman is supported by the « os coccyx » barely touching the cushion, and this position resembles « The Herculean Feat » (No. 23), but is much less tiring. A very supple-bodied female will not need to put her legs round the man's body, crossing them behind his back, but will lift them up on to his shoulders. The prick enters well within when her knees are under his armpits, but bores still further into her vagina in the last manner I have just described, but which is more fatiguing and can only be realised with a young and flexible — jointed female — a ballet girl for instance.

48 Waste Not, Want Not

The woman lies on her back on die bed, her thighs as open as possible so that the knees are drawn up almost touching her nipples. The man mounts upon her, placing her calves on his shoulders, to keep her legs and thighs uplifted. He pushes his piercer into the cunt which is well exposed ready for his thrusts and is gaping open. As he drives backwards and forwards to satisfy her lubricity, he leans the weight of his shoulders on her calves each time he shoves his drill into the hairy chasm. Each shove of his arse drives his manly staff yet a little more in. Meanwhile he caresses all her charms, and his happy victim feels the darling prick touching her very soul, and, when about to discharge, the man should make no backward movement, but remain buried to the root and thus his throbbing cock plugs completely up the entrance and prevents the spunk that spurts into her vitals flowing out again. His partner should press forward, opening herself as much as she can to receive his burning offering and spend herself at the same time. Not a single drop is lost by this method.

49 The Grand Entrance

The woman is seated in the edge of a sofa, her thighs open, the knees well back and uplifted, her legs bent under so that her heels touch her buttocks, and her toes are supported by cushions piled up until on a level with the sofa. A pillow is behind her for her back to lean upon. The man goes down on his knees between the cushions on which her feet rest. He approaches the place of worship where his advent is impatiently expected and plunges in until their two bushes become as one, putting his hands underneath the lady's arse, to draw her towards him, while at the same time he lunges and retreats with all the strength of his loins. Their faces meet: and so do their quivering tongues, while both her marble bum and his brawny arse join in the dance. Soon the fire of pleasure burns with intensity and their mutual and copious gushes of lustful quintessence prove, by the excess of salacious joy experienced, the merit of this fascinating posture, called with truth « The Grand Entrance », as the two folding doors of the femine laboratory as naturally completely open.

(Here the dialogue, which has been more or less a monologue, was interrupted by the entrance of the punctual charwoman, heralded by a timid honeymoon knock at the door. It was six o'clock and she brought the dinner, and laid the cloth. During the repast, the conversation became uninteresting on account of the presence of the faithful « slavey ». whom it was unnecessary to scandalise, although she knew perfectly well the extent of the understanding that reigned between Charlie and Maud. When appetite was satisfied, the old woman cleared everything away, but did not forget to leave on the table another clean service, some cold viands, wine, spirits and mineral waters, for fear the lovers should feel inclined to pick a little bit before retiring for the night, and she disappeared with strict orders not to trouble unless she heard the bell. The door bolted, Maud reclined upon the sofa and, summoning her lover, begged him, to continue the subject he had let drop when dinner was served. Charlie, as usual, wanted but very little asking and started again to finish the lecture that so excited his mistress)

DIALOGUE IV

50 The Donkey Ride

This is a very amusing manner, but it is not everybody who can carry it out successfully. You must first get a donkey, not too obstinate, and the lovers must have some idea of how to ride these capricious beasts without being frightened, and the woman must mount like a man. In these bicycling days there should be no difficulty about so small a matter. The woman cocks her leg over the donkey's back, where there is no saddle, only a rug, and a pair of shortened stirrups. If the spot chosen for this randy ride is not secluded enough for the cavalier and his lady to be completely naked, the female must lift up her petticoats back and front, lean forward encircling the donkey's neck with both her arms, throwing up her arse by rising in the stirrups. The man mounts behind her, leans back, holding on the donkey's tail with one hand, while with the other he slips his cock into the loving cunt dog-fashion which, by the position she is now in, is easy enough. When all is ready, the woman, empaled, drops down between her fucker's thighs, and her lover catches hold of the animal's tail with both his hands behind him. Now they dig their knees into the donkey's sides, which starts him off and at the same time holds them fast in the postures they have chosen. The donkey trots and shakes their backsides well right and left. That movement increases their pleasure and, when they are about to spend, the lover pulls the ass's tail, which finally causes him to kick out behind, or jib, however patient by nature he may be, forcing the man's prick to penetrate still further, to the great and certain voluptuous satisfaction of both parties. But they must not lose their head when they lose their cream, as it sometimes happens, for then the jibbing beast gets rid of his double burden and the lovers find themselves on the ground with all their spendings knocked out of them.

51 The Gunner and the Cannon

The woman lies on her back and loins; arse, thighs and legs outside the bed and across it man stands in front of her, taking one of her feet in each hand just above the ankle and holds them up as high as possible, a trifle forward, but straight up and open. He can thus take a proper view of the breech and point his rammer to clean the cannon. He pushes his prick forward and by his position it should slip in by itself. Once within, he shoves on with might and main, at the same time thrusting up and down one or the other of the legs he holds, or both together, which causes all sorts of varied motions to be felt inside the cunt, not for getting nippings and rubbings which voluptuously excite the thrice happy prick, making it stiffer than ever, and communicating to the two working partners indescribable pleasure, which finishes — alas! but too soon — by a double reciprocal ejaculation.

52 How to Get a Boy

The woman lies on her back on the bed across it, her legs outside. The man stands up in front of her and takes up her right leg at the calf, placing it under his left arm. With his right he lifts up the left leg of the woman, which he places straight up the calf reaching thus to the front of the right shoulder, at the side of his face. With one hand he opens the lips of the eager woman's lower mouth, plants his prick inside and shoves away with his arse until he spends, being careful to first try and time himself so as to ejaculate at the same moment as the female, and secondly to drive his emitting cock in as far as his strength will permit, so that not the least drop precious liquor shall he lost. The opinion of several learned doctors, specialists for the generative organs, is that to get a boy the woman must have the right side lower than the left when being fucked, so that the man's seed should fall towards the right flank, where they opine male children are always conceived.

53 How to Get a Girl

This is the same posture, only the man tucks under his right arm the left thigh of the female. Then with his left hand the lifts the woman's right leg straight up, so that her right side is higher than the left. The rest as in the preceding position, where I have explained the idea of the learned authorities. It results from these two postures, and from the reasons given, that we might attain the same result in many different ways of fucking (« The Ordinary », « The Inseparables », Nos. 1 and 2, or any other where the woman lies on her back; her arse uplifted by cushions or a pillow), as long as we do not forget that, where the birth of a boy is desired, the woman should have her left side higher than the right and « vice versa », if she yearns to bring yet another cunt into the world, to delight the butterfly rogerer who flits from flower, tasting the honey of each. There can never too many cunts on this earth!

54 The Living Mattress

The man lies on his back stretched out at full length on the bed, his prick stiff standing like Nelson's monument. The woman mounts upon him and takes her place as in the « Empalement Backwards », (No. 20). When she has herself lodged the column in its nook, she stretches out her thighs on those of her companion and leans backwards, reclining with her shoulders upon his chest, and she turns her face towards him a little to give and receive lascivious kisses. Thus she rests as upon a mattress, and the man, his tongue between her lips, presses her titties, her belly, the bushy mount and the clitoris, passing his hands from behind over her sweet body. They move gently and cautiously, as with heavy strokes the prick might slip from its prison, as in this posture it does not advance very far into the cunt, where the woman can, however, keep it in its place with her hand. To perform properly thus a long prick is needful and a fellow boasting such a weapon will have no need to fear injuring his mistress.

55 The Toad

The woman lies on her back at full length on the bed, a large pillow or even two under her arse to force the cunt well up in front; her head and shoulders are also supported by cushions. (In Scotland, I believe, the heavy family bible is often made use of in this posture — a favourite one across the border). The man gets over her in ordinary fashion. When he is in, the woman lifts up her legs and thighs as high as she can, keeping them well open, so that her heels touch her buttocks above the line of her thighs. Her knees press against her lover, near his armpits. They are pressed together in each other's arms, and the man profits by the position of the woman, who in this way presents her cunt as open as possible, to stove in his tool till their bushes mingle. With many a groan and sigh of lust, with repeated strokes of loins and arse they enjoy transports of erotic joy which do not last for ever and shortly a double emission brings down the essence of love.

56 The Basket

A round bottomless basket is suspended by its two handles to a cord running over a strong pulley, or ship's « block », which is fixed to the ceiling, the end of the rope reaching the ground. The woman sits in the basket between the handles, her back supported by one side, and her legs thrown over the other, hanging over the edge, which comes under her knees. Her arses ticks out of the bottomless basket and her mount and cunt are forced out as well. The man draws the basket up a little by pulling the rope and lies down at full length under it, his shoulders on the ground and his prick upstanding like Cleopatra's favourite needle, facing the secret beauties of the woman which pout between her arse-cheeks. He lets the basket gently down again, holding the rope with one hand to keep the load at a proper height, and with the other he adjusts his prick in the cunt. As soon as he is landed, he pulls the basket up and down alternately and gradually, so as not to let his cock slip out, and when it is a prisoner root and all, he can give a hall-turn to the basket the left or right, which deliciously twists his prick, makes it as hard and as a piece of wood and procures incalculable pleasure to the lovers, obliging them to discharge as if their sexual organs were spermatic fountains.

57 Upright Fucking

This is the counterpart of « Dog-Fashion Upright » (No. 38). The lovers are face to face; the woman mounting upon a low stool, or cushions, arranged in such a manner that her cunt is on a level with the man's prick, who gets into her in that position. He holds her to him with one hand, their mouths glued together, her heaving breasts crushed against his hairy chest. With his other hand, he directs his cock and, once inside, clasps her by the arse to draw her close to his body. Now they both agitate their frames in unison, lip-licking and tongue-sucking, crushed close together, and rubbing their two skins one against the other. They are soon compelled to finish as usual, by a mutual ecstatic discharge. This posture is not a very comfortable one, and « Dog-Fashion Upright » (No. 38) is no easier. They are both tiring, requiring long pricks to give much pleasure, and can only be recommended for an occasional momentary whim.

58 The Game of Honey-pots

The concluding remarks of the last posture apply to this one, which demands a long prick, although analogous to « Waste Not, Want Not », (No. 48), and « The Grand Entrance », (No. 49), which are far from being so difficult. The one I am about to describe requires the couple to be flexible and adroit, without sufficient reward awaiting them for their pains; the same pleasure being procurable in other ways less fatiguing and easy for all. Thus it may be only noted for being a simple curiosity, to be tried once in a while. The woman lies on her back on the bed or on a soft carpet; her loins supported by a cushion. She lifts up her thighs, keeping them well open, so that her knees come up to her nipples and her heels touch her buttocks. When she is thus squatting, on her hams, the man straddles across her, his feet outside to the right and left of her body, the part of his arse at the function of his thighs placed upon the insteps of the woman, who forces herself to take up as little space as possible. He insinuates his tool through the four thighs into the lady's cunt, passing his arms round and between her knees and body to grasp her arse and draw her to him. She, on her side, holds him by the neck and advances her rosy mouth for their tongues to meet. When the man is comfortably installed, he moves up and down without any rough movements, so as not to let his cock escape from the grip of the hairy lips, and everything finishes by a double and copious outburst, well-earned by the dificulty vanquished in succeding this posture, so inconvenient for both.

59 The Swing

A bench about two feet long, well-cushioned, is fixed by each end to a long double rope, knotted and plaited together about three feet above. The ropes are fixed to trees, or to a beam, so as to form a swing. The man sits in the middle of the seat of the swing; the woman places herself across him, as in « The Cock-Horse », (No. 39), and puts his prick in the proper place, passing her thighs round him so that her legs are crossed behind his back. Each of the actors clasps hold of the cords to left and right and the man starts the swing with one foot on the ground to begin with, and afterwards keeps it going by the movements of his arse and loins, generously returned by the woman, which posess the double property of accelerating the swinging diversion and being exactly needful to help the fucking which our lovers are having while passing through the air. It is prudent that they should pass a belt round their bodies attached at each end to the cords of the swing, for without this precaution, in the moment of enjoyment, when all strength leaves them and their eyes grow dim, they may chance to let go the rope, and fall heavily to the ground. The woman, although the most ardent, is at bottom the weakest, and she should on no account be allowed to spend on a swing without being fastened to it. Ederly voluntary cuckolds, who allow their wives to have a lover on condition that they be present when he is fucking their better half, will do well to have the operation performed on the swing on a summer afternoon. They can look up and enjoy the sight of united cock and cunt flying through the air above their nose. In the case of a fall, the impotent husband can leave off frigging himself, and catch one or the other or both, if they tumble off and thus will have done something useful for once in his life.

60 The Swinging Target

The woman sits on the swing alone, on the edge, lifting up her legs and opening her thighs, pressing her heels to her buttocks, so as to reduce her hody, so to speak, to the smallest possible compass and presenting her cunt outside the seat of the swing. She leans her head and shoulders well back, thus forcing the private parts still more forward and holds on tightly to the ropes. The man stands in front of her, prick in hand, pointing to the centre of the living target. He is soon ensconced in the hairy bulls-eye and with a slight push drives the swing from him. As it returns with its laughing, lascivious burden he takes good aim and should land within at every return of the swing. He continues this play as long as it pleases him, and, when he feels the venereal spasm approaching, he seizes the opportunity to stop the swing and discharge at his ease while the lady, tired of the oscillation, invites osculation and mixes her essence with his.

61 The Double-Headed Beast; or, Two Ends to the Stick

The woman lies at full length on the bed, sideways, presenting her back to the man who takes the same position but in a double-reversed sense. That is to say he is on his back, on the opposite side to that of the woman, his head towards her tail. He passes one leg and thigh between hers, below her posterior beauties; his other is thrown over her, thus bringing his bust towards hers on a level with their groins. Now is the time to adjust the cock, by bending it into the woman's cunt and keeping it in the warm and moist furrow with one hand, which also tickles the clitoris and the mount within reach, while both push on, retreat and push again, but with great care, so as not to break the connection. For this is yet another of those postures requiring skill, precaution, and above all a long lithe prick, with which there is of course always a better chance of succeeding no matter whether the position be easy or difficult If you don't believe me, ask the ladies! With a long prick it is very easy to take a few inches off the wrong end by not letting the whole of the monster rush right in, but what remedy is there for a short cock? It is impossible to add an extra joint.

62 The Sack of Corn Forwards

The woman lies across the bed on her back. She up her legs and thighs, and right and left passes her feet in two loops of a rope, sufficiently high up so that she is only supported on the sheets by her head and shoulders and her loins, hips and all the rest are opened out and in the air. The man gets on the bed and passes his head and his body, from front to back, between the open thighs of the lady, to whom he presents his arse, while her head is between his feet He leans forwards, fixes his prick in her cleft and, once ensconced, he lies quite forward, supports his hands on the bed near her shoulder-blades, and she can enjoy the view in perspective of the muscles on his brawny arse and his heavy bag and balls, agitated by the erotic exercise he is taking. His thrust is soon quicken, driven on by the play of his dear sweetheart's deft digits, unable to resist the desire to tickle his appendages and slap the cheeks of his posteriors, stretched close to her eyes. The man fucks, and caresses and moulds all the backside beauties that his eyes devour, and he can even pass his hands in front to visit the heaving snowy breasts and other beauties with easy distance. The final result of all this refined debauchery is a magnificent ejaculation, of which not a drop is lost for the lady, as by this position all the allowance runs to the very bottom of the womb, tickling deliciously this most sensitive organ.

63 The Sack of Corn Backwards

This is the contrary of the preceding position. The woman is placed as before, but the man, instead of getting between her thighs from front to back, takes up his position now from back to front and consequently plants his stake dog-fashion, having his feet behind the shoulders of the woman on the bed. He leans forward, his face resting on her breasts which he can kiss, lick and rub his nose against. In return, the woman can advance her randy mouth and tongue and lifting herself up a little suck his breath. The battle terminates by a volley from both parties and they have as much pleasure as in the preceding posture. In both these methods of fucking, the man truly resembles a sack of corn placed on a trestle — that idea furnishing the titles to the two positions I have just described and which terminate the salacious series.

Charlie (stopping). — I think now that I have finished my task as far as regards the 1st § of the 1st Section of my 1st Chapter. The longest and most difficult is done, but it is now ten o'clock; I am a little tired through talking so long, so let us to bed, so that I may rest in your arms. I suppose that you are not visiting me with the sole idea of listening to my talk. Your letter promised me a day and two nights of love and passion. You must keep your word. My lecture on the diverse moves of sacrificing to Venus must not cause my darling to perjure herself.

Maud. — Wicked man! I expect you want to try and realise a few living pictures with me, copied from some of the lewd canvasses you have unrolled just now. I consent, but promise me that, after a few hours of pleasure, you will continue your enchanting dissertations, which interest me so much that I don't intend to sleep a wink until after you have thoroughly exhausted the subject, even though I set up listening to you the whole night long.

Charlie. — You know well that your will is law for me, But first to bed! [The lovers retire between the sheets and they try a few experiments, realising a respectable number of the foregoing postures, and then Charlie, faithful to his word, continues his sermon on the mount., (of Venus), as if he had not sustained the delightful interruption].

DIALOGUE V

§ II

SODOMY WITH WOMEN

Charlie. — I have finished the description of the various methods used to fuck a woman in the natural orifice, and I now come to a few other ways. An old song says :

« The distance between a girl's cunt and arse-hole,
Is but a foul crabs' jump without vaulting pole »

This being mathematically incontestable, we must conclude therefore that all the postures I have already described can serve nearly all just as well for sodomising a woman as for rogering her. But although a woman is cunt all over for a true fucker, the act of sodomy or buggering, even with the feminine sex, should only be a momentary caprice for him and not a leading habitual vice. The sodomite in general is right up to a certain point when he maintains that all tastes exist in nature and the best of all is our particular one, whichever it may be. But it is none the less logical to say that, if all men had this exclusive propensity for spending in the woman's arse, the world would come to an end. This motive alone shows the dangerous trap into which we should fall if we allowed such principles to be indefinitely applied. They are true at bottom, if you will, as this limitless extension would soon bring about a radical solution of the problem of depopulation. But happily there are a very small number of exclusive sodomites, in proportion to the considerably stronger army of old-fashioned cunt-fuckers, so that there is very little harm done and we need not trouble about the question. Let everyone do as he or she likes, as long as strict secrecy is kept, without scandal, or moral and physical violence. I frankly confess that is has always seemed pitiful to me to drawn arguments from religious law against pederastic pleasure. I go further and. declare that religion has nothing to do with fucking in any shape or form whatsoever, if quietly carried out as I said just now. I am at liberty to speak freely as I am a perfectly disinterested party, this peculiar taste never having been mine. I have perforated a few blushing backsides, I confess, out of pure, or rather impure, wayward fancy, and curiosity, with women only. Some of the sweet innocents have even begged me to distend their wrinkled sepia, factory, either because they wanted to try the experiment, or as they told me, for fear of getting that swelling behind the navel that rarely goes down under nine months. But I have always preferred the true road to paradise and I think it is rank blasphemy to mix up our bibles and prayers in all these fucking follies. When will the common anserous herd, as credulous as they are silly and addle-headed, clear their muddy brains and cease to listen as if they were oracles, to certain individuals of different religious denominations, who are not such fools as they look and who mix up, or more truly « feign » to mix up, so-calleds acred decrees with sociabye-laws and sentiments of true morality, the only ones that nature inspires man with at his birth, with the repugnancies that the prejudices of conventional education alone bestow on simple and timid minds! These gentry who preach from acting as they talk and, when together with their colleagues, they do not fail to unmask and agree that everything is generally permissible when no one is hurt. They do not stop even there when it comes to the application, as they admit without restriction that nothing is forbidden if it is hidden. But enough of such serious argument. I am getting too oserious and my theme is a gay one. Let me return to my bottoms. Nearly all the postures for cunt-fucking can be used for buggering a woman, by reason of the neighbourhood of the two apertures. To my knowledge there exists no way of bottom-piercing that cannot also be used for copulation in front and, as I believe I have described every possible way of plugging a cunt, it would be going over the same ground again to explain them all once more as applied to sodomy with your enchanting sex. Let it suffice for me to tell you that in all the postures described as for the cunt, it is only necessary to place the mans cock a few inches higher or lower according to the position of the woman for her to be fucked in the arse, as the two holes are so near to each other that the realisation of the attitudes is just as easy and the change of lodging is indifferent for the action in itself.

Nevertheless the easiest ways to get up a lady's fundament are those which I have described in the cunt-postures under the name of : The Back-View (No. 7). — The Elastic Woman (No. 14). — The Wheelbarrow Backwards (No. 18). — Empalement Backwards (No. 20). — The Basket (No. 56). — The

Sack of Corn Backwards (No. 63), and all the dog-fashion postures : No. 11, 18, 20, 25, 27, 29, 32. 32, 33, 34, 35, 36, 37, 38. 43, 45, 46, 48, and 53.

The remarks I have made here and there, concerning the facility or difficulty of execution of the various postures, apply-equally, sometimes more and sometimes less, to their performance in sodomitical style with women.

It must also not be forgotten that in all cases and in all ways of sodomising the female, it is the mans duty to take up his position in such a manner that one of his hands can frig her cunt, although his prick neglects it, tickling the clitoris, the nipples, etc. The entrance, too, should never be effected with brutality or violence and, until the little brown hole is sufficiently dilated to admit the prick easily, a little grease should always be applied and the masculine acorn will be all the more comfortable if anointed also before the Socratic act. A very pretty preparation before inserting, the battering-ram in the back precints is a simple kiss or warm caress of a moist tongue, when the saliva takes the place of cold-cream. Indeed, this voluptuous kiss is generally well received by both sexes, even when no pederastic violence is intended.

To sum up, men should never be selfish or ungrateful; we ought to try to give as much pleasure as we can while we are receiving voluptuous joy from the woman, and the feeling that we are doing our duty to our companion will double our lubricity.

SECTION II

POSTURES WITHOUT INTRODUCTION OF THE VIRIL MEMBER, BUT MUTUALLY VOLUPTUOUS; RECIPROCAL FRIGGING AND GAMAHUCHING

You can well understand that these postures are not very numerous, as it would be idle to describe all the ways and means by which a loving couple can mutually frig; seated, standing, lying, down, forward, backward, etc. For the woman one or more fingers of her lover will suffice, or his hand will rummage her mount and cunt, tickling her clitoris, the large outer lips and the smaller inner ones, the perineum, the arse-hole, the breasts and their nipples, the posteriors, the shoulders, the back and loins, etc. To please man the woman also uses her hands to grasp, shake stroke and caress her lover's prick and balls, the neutral ground between his hairy purse and arse-hole, which later retreat also comes in for a good share of tickling, not forgetting the cheeks of his bum, etc... The whole to he accompanied with reciprocal kisses on every part of the body, dove-like slobbering with tongues entwined and all other ordinary episodes.

The best and principal methods for mutual masturbation I shall now describe, remarking that all other means are only copied or derived from them.

1 The Genuine Frig

The man is seated on a sofa, by the side of the woman, on her right hand. She is seated too. He puts his left arm round her waist or passes it over or under her left shoulder to mould her breasts, or slips it under her arse to press her bottom. With his right hand, he gently opens the lips of her cunt and tickles her clitoris with one finger, pushing it in and out and round about in every direction. To increase the pleasure he must moisten his thumb and middle-finger with a little saliva and, pressing the thumb on the clitoris, slip the index into the cunt and the middle-finger into the arse-hole, bending the other digits. He rapidly and lightly moves his fingers thus placed, forwards and backwards, gently at first and furiously fast when the discharge is near. His nails should he cut short and well filed and all fugged edges rounded off, as a scratch might do great harm to the delicate internal parts of the woman's genitals, leading to the formation of sores in the whomb and rectum. The woman on her side takes her lovers prick in her right hand and shakes it softly and voluptuously. She uncovers the sensitive nut by drawing down the foreskin and pulls up the hood again, gently at first and then quicker tightening her grasp so as to stretch the « fraenum » by drawing down the skin of the prick towards the root. She lets her hand travel softly down towards the root, and then comes back to the gland, wetting her thumb in her mouth and passing it backwards and forwards over the fraenum and the ruby head, which she lightly rubs.

During this time, her left hand is busy with her lover's balls. She presses them with a loving soft grasp, caressing the bag and its contents and the root of the prick, the perineum and its vicinity, etc. She also can wet a finger of the left hand too, and tickle his arse-hole, and if she can, force it right up his fundament.

The couple embrace and kiss at the same time, pressing against each other; they do battle with their tongues and soon the burning spunk bursts reciprocally from the reservoirs, inundating their active hands.

2 The Strawberries

The woman lies on her back on a bed or sofa, her knees lifted up a little and well apart. The man places himself at the right of the couch near her, seated, or on his knees, according to the height of the piece of furniture in use. He passes his left arm round his charmers neck and brings it above her chest, grasps her left breast and tickles the strawberry nipple with one of his fingers. At the same time, by stooping a trifle, he takes in his mouth the corresponding strawberry of the right bubby, causing the stiffened point of his tongue to quiver on and about it. His right hand, the fingers duly moistened, slips under the uplifted thighs of the lady, and the thumb is on the magic button, the index in the vagina and the middle digit up the tiny dark hole. From time to time the lover abandons the right nipple, to fasten his lips to hers and tickle her tongue with his. She, to please him in return, passes her right hand between his body and the bed and catches hold of his prick, frigging it well and also its appendages, with all due science, gentleness and with fairy-like touches, using all the little tricks and dodges described in the foregoing frig, so as to properly caress him who is caressing her so well himself. The conclusion is imminent and is marked by a delicious reciprocal spend which the lovers exchange in their hands with the utmost satisfaction.

Besides frigging, there are other means for enjoying mutual pleasure between the sexes without the intromission of the viril organ, so much feared by many women who have not even confidence in French letters, or the little sponge, and still less in the solemn oath taken by the lover to withdraw at the critical moment and not spend inside. I allude to gamahuching, name that is given to the action of tickling, sucking and licking with the tongue and mouth the sexual parts of man or woman.

Here is the description :

3 Sixty-Nine

The woman lies on her back on the bed, her thighs apart, her knees uplifted. The man straddles over her in the contrary sense, on his knees, her head being between his thighs. He stretches out to his full length, the elbows supported on the bed at the side of her hips and his face is hidden between her thighs. He passes his hands under her posteriors to open the lips of her cunt and place his mouth upon it, putting his stiffened tongue on the clitoris and frisking the point all round it. He must plunge his tongue as far as he can into the interior of the cunt, sucking the clitoris and drawing it up between his lips, while with the index in the vagina and the middle-finger up the arse, he shoves backwards and forwards, caressing and stroking all the other parts with his other hand. During this time the woman has been active. With one hand she has popped his sugar-stick into her mouth, nibbling it, sucking it, tickling the fraenum and ruby head with her pointed tongue, holding the foreskin tightly back. With her other hand she tickles, caresses, presses and dandles the balls, the root of the prick that is not entirely in her mouth, his hairs, the perineum, the arse-hole, into which she forces a moistened finger, and the arse-cheeks which she softly strokes, and gently pinches and slaps. These caresses are continued until the approach of the culminating pleasure, when it seems as if the woman was trying to swallow the prick, so much does she force it down her throat while madly sucking at it, while the man is evidently trying to press his whole face into her cunt and eat her saucy clitoris, so much does he press inside the former and draw the latter between his lips and teeth. Thus each of the lovers receives in his mouth the spunk of the other without quitting their position until the discharge is complete and all the reservoirs are dry, swallowing or rejecting afterwards, according to their taste or their passion of a moment, the divine liquid so voluptuously and salaciously emitted.

This position is always known as « Sixty-Nine » from the position of the lovers' heads, as they form exactly the two figures 69, showing a head whichever way they are turned. The sign of the Zodiac ; « Libra » the Balance, offers the same appearance.

4 Sixty-Nine Reversed

This is the same posture « vice versa » the only difference being that the man is now lying on his back, the knees drawn up a little, and the woman mounts upon him, on her knees, right and left of his head, her cunt on his face and her arse in the air, while she has her head between his thighs sucking his prick while he licks her cunt. The rest as in the preceding explanation; the climax being the same, so that there is nothing more to tell you of the original game of heads and tails.

5 Combined Gamahuching and Breast-Fucking

The man sits in the middle of a low sofa, and in front of him, at his feet, between his open legs is a stool. He leans a little backwards, the loins and shoulders supported by some cushions. The woman mounts upon the sofa, turning her bottom towards the mans face, and, placing her feet upon the couch, she stoops forward and leans her hands upon the stool in front of her between his legs. By this position, being opened out and leaning forward, she offers her cunt below her posteriors fully exposed and outstretched to the mans mouth. He clasp his lips to the hairy slit, his tongue quivering inside it and licking the clitoris, and he kisses her round bum and also the arse-hole, not forgetting to push his tongue therein — a soft caress not to be forgotten — and when he is sucking with all his might the throbbing cunt, he can also let his nose press against the backside. By the way the lovers are now placed the breasts of the woman are touching the man's prick. He puts it between the two heaving globes and passing his arms between her legs presses with both hands, so that the titties close upon his cock.

Working with arse and loins as well as sucking her cunt, he soon sets the woman frisking and moving convulsively about beneath his caresses, and it is not long before the man receives in his mouth the liquid proof of her enjoyment which he returns with interest between her breasts.

6 The Man Sat Upon

The man lies on the bed, crossways a little, his knees up, the heels touching the buttocks, turned towards the inside of the bed, his head on the outside edge. The woman places a stool near his face, mounts upon it, with one foot, passing the other over her lover and placing him and bending down, she supports her cunt on his face and her arse comes upon his chest, just below his neck. She does not press too heavily so as not to stifle him and lifts herself up a little on her feet, putting one hand upon his head which is supported by the edge of the bed. Stretching out her other hand she takes a firm grasp of his cock and frigs him cleverly, tickling his balls, the neutral ground between his bag and arse-hole and the root of the prick, following up by a gentle rubbing of the sensitive scarlet bead, drawing the foreskin backwards and forwards. The man, with one hand passed behind her, plays with her arse, which is turned towards his feet and supports the robust posteriors on his mouth, while his tongue tickles the clitoris and plunges into the vagina as in the preceding sucking sketches. He passes his other hand between her body and the leg that is outstretched and supported by the stool, bringing it round in front to part the hairs and the lips of the cunt, so as to make the vibrating gap more accessible to his greedy mouth. Lastly, he strokes the randy woman's belly and feels her bubbies, and in deep gratitude she lets loose her spending essence over his face and in his mouth, and he, far from ungrateful, shows his sympathy by spunking vigorously into the soft white palm which is frigging him.

7 Heads and Tails

The couple lie upon the ground in the position of « Sixty-Nine Reversed », (No. 4 « ante »). When all is ready, the man puts the woman's thighs over his shoulders, right and left, and, holding them firmly, gets up standing, the woman encircling his loins with her arms. When they are thus upright, the woman has her head downwards and her legs up in the air. She takes the stiff cock in her mouth, holding on with one hand to the loins of the man standing firm on his feet and her other hand serves to tickle his balls, etc., as in the other gamahuching bouts. The man pressing the woman, whose cunt and arse-hole are close to his mouth, to him by one hand on the small of her back, passes his other hand over her backside, parting her bush and the cunny-lips, working his tongue within it according to the gamahuching maxims already laid down. The same hand is next needed to caress her bum and its wrinkled hole, etc., until feeling the sovereign pleasure about to manifest itself, and his strength leaving him in consequence, he backs towards the bed and falls thereon so as to discharge in comfort and without fear of accident.

8 A Lazy Sixty-Nine

This is the game of « Sixty-Nine » (No. 3 « ante ») or « Sixty-Nine Reversed » (No. 4); but now the lovers try it both lying full length on the side, the man being on the right side and the woman lies doing « Sixty-Nine » with him on the right side also. Or else the man is on his left side and the woman also, but always in the « Sixty-Nine » position, so that in any case she has her cunt near his mouth and his cock is pointed towards her rosy lips. Each lilts the thigh up a little, on the opposite side to that which he or she is lying, so as to facilitate the passage of the others face between the thighs, as well as the hands which exert themselves in caressing stokes, pats and pinches all round within reach, while their two mouths do their mutual duty to the sexual parts. The lovers have thus no weight to support. All is pleasure without any trouble, increasing their joy and making them spend in each other's mouth with more voluptuousness than ever.

I think, my darling, that you are now fully instructed in all the postures that two lovers can take if they wish to exhaust all the delights of love without dangerous penetrations, which might lead to living proofs of adultery and fornication, but in which nevertheless the pleasure is mutual and partaken of by both, and the enjoyment of the final melting moment of spending transport is complete for lover and mistress.

Do now I will pass on to the pleasures of the man alone, by the aid of the woman without the latter taking any share in the fun, except by the innate knowledge of the pleasure she gives. For it is also a great enjoyment to give pleasure to the loved one and note the effect our efforts produce, even when we do not perhaps experience the actual spasm. But it is none the less agreeable to make the object of our adoration spend freely, even if we do not discharge at the same time, although there is no law to prevent us frigging ourselves while showering voluptuous caress of hand and tongue on another.

CHAPTER II

PLEASURES OF MAN ALONE, BY THE AID OF WOMAN, BUT WITHOUT HER RECIPROCAL PARTICIPATION

1 The False Fuck

The woman is tired of spending, but the man is still clamorous for more. She lies on her side and so does the man behind her. He approaches his body and slips his prick between her thighs, which close upon it and he gravely fucks between her snowy columns as if he was in her cunt or arse-hole. To heighten the illusion he plays with, and feels, all her charms and she, twisting her face half round towards him, gives him her randy tongue, while she tightens her thighs and moves them gently together to excite by the touch of their smooth skin the emprisoned prick, which rubs against the hair of her cunt, while the white, round, velvety arse warms the mans belly. Such a combination of caresses soon forces his amorous sluices to burst and the inside of her thighs is soon sticky with the jet of his manly essence, position can be recommended to all having to do with very young girls or half-virgins. The same remark applies in nearly every to all easy postures where no actual penetration is required. Incestuous papas please note.

2 Real Suck

The man is half seated on a sofa or bed. The woman goes down on her knees before him, seizing his sugar-stick in one hand and placing it in her mouth. She sucks it at her ease, while with her other hand she tickles, presses and dandles the balls with every accompaniment and salacious play before described and which it is idle to repeat at each change of position. The man can always find some mischief for his idle hands to do in pressing her hubbies and other charms within his reach until the shell bursts in the warm, soft mouth of the sucking, licking, slobbering, half-choked darling.

She must not cease the sweet play of her caressing tongue and lips and teeth round the shaft, and swollen red head of the bursting prick, until she is sure that the last drop has exuded from the orifice of the urethra, and the true sucking female, she who really enjoys having a cock in her mouth, excited by the taste, the perfume, its excitable movements, the warning throbbings and final heavenly explosion of seminal liquor, eagerly swallows the entire dose, and I may say that the lady who keeps it all in the hollow of her cheeks till she can conveniently get rid of it by expectorating into a convenient receptacle, is unworthy of the name of a true British sweet sucker.

3 Bag-Piping

The man stands up, his backside supported by the edge of the bed and the woman is on her knees before him, either on the ground or on a pile of cushions according to her height. She places the beloved prick between her two breasts, the point coming under her chin, and she presses her two full globes with each hand, looking with sweet adoration at her lover, who is moving his arse as if he was in her cunt or her bottom. His weapon thus pressed between the bubbies, which also rub against his balls, is deliciously titillated and soon a superb jet of seed spurts from the dark red swelling acorn, bespattering the neck and face of the woman and falling back upon her bust. To enjoy this pastime fully it is needless to say that the woman must have enough development of the breasts to be able to press them against the manly organ as if they were the two bags of a pair of bag-pipes : hence the name given to his method of spending. Some cold-cream between the breasts will be found an improvement. With a little skill and wish to please, the lady can bend down her head and tickle the top of the prick with her tongue and, if she really loves the man who is thus boldly fucking her titties, she will open wide her mouth to receive the fountain of seminal liquid upon her lips and tongue.

4 Bag-Piping Reversed

This is the same pleasurable exercice for the male, but with a few extra salacious novelties added.

The woman lies on her back on a low bench or narrow couch, her head reaching just at the edge. The man straddles across her face, his arse just touching her chin and she has a good view of his posteriors, his brown hole, etc. He is standing up, his legs to the right and left of her body and face. He places his prick between the breasts, the point towards her navel, and presses the heaving globes with his two hands thus manufacturing a delicious cunt for himself, into which he pushes as if it was the real article. While he moves, rubbing his prick between the fleshy hillocks, the woman kisses and licks his arse, the perineum, and the arse-hole which is so near her face, pushing in her pointed tongue as well, or a moistened finger; not forgetting to pet and dandle his balls with her hands which she passes behind her lover. These lewd gymnastics soon make him discharge, sprinkling the stomach, belly and navel of his darling with a cascade of essence which runs down to the mount and the cunt.

5 A Ride in the Valley

This is almost the same as « Bag-Piping (No. 3 « ante »), as far as the result is concerned. The woman lies at full length on a narrow bench or couch and the man cocks his leg over her face, standing up, one leg to the left and the other to the right, his face turned towards hers. He puts his prick in the valley of her breasts, between the two proud white globes and she presses them together to form an imitation cunt. His hands are free to play with all the charms he can reach; he tickles the nipples on the bubbles that emprison his prick and, passing his arms, behind, trifles with her belly and the hair on her mount; the climax coming eventually and causing an inundation of spunk upon the neck and lace of his delighted sweetheart.

6 Armpit Fucking

The woman bends one knee to the ground and the man stands before her. She puts his prick under her armpit between her body and the top of her plump arm, either from behind or from the front. She squeezes the prick against her side and the man moves as if in a cunt. He feels her bubbies and she softly wriggles her arm, while holding the man's arse with one hand, if he is facing her. She caresses his muscular backside, slapping it and tickling the division of the cheeks, pushing a wetted linger in the hole in the middle. With the other hand, she strokes the balls and the perineum as well as the root of the prick, which soon, unable to support the sensation and all these caresses any longer, spurts out a tremendous volley of generative fluid on the back, loins and arse of the women. If the man has taken up his position behind the woman, the woman cannot lavish all these tender touches upon him; she can only react the end of his prick with her free hand and play with the scarlet top which comes from behind and appears in front of her body from under the hairy armpit. In this case he finishes this whimsical way of enjoyment by spending in her hand.

7 Imitation Sodomy

The man is seated on the edge of a chair, his body well forward. The woman approaches him, backwards, presenting her arse. She leans forward, supported by the back of another chair. Her posteriors thus nicely jutted out in front of the man, he puts his prick in the crack of her arse, between its two full cheeks; his balls being near the end of her cunt. He presses her bottom with his two hands, to make this randy gutter as narrow as possible. The woman moves lewdly about and he shoves heartily up and down till the boiling liquor bursts forth, as a consequence of these libidinous caresses, inundating the loins and arse of the woman, trickling down the division of the cheeks of the bottom, which form an elegant imitation cunt for a prentice pederast.

CHAPTER III

FEMALE PLEASURE BY THE AID OF THE MAN, BUT WITHOUT RECIPROCITY

1 The Selfish Gamahuche

The woman places herself on a pedestal, the shaft of a column, or a light small piece of furniture, such as a night-table, on which there is just room enough for her arse. At either side hangs a rope, which she grasps, and throws herself backwards, seated on the edge of the pedestal so that her « os coccyx » alone supports her body. By this her arse and cunt are thrown well forward; her legs and thighs are wide open and her feet are placed left and right on the backs of two chairs standing at each side of her table. Thus her knees are bent up to her breasts and the man goes down on his knees between the chairs and her open thighs. He presses his mouth to the cunt so prettily offered and exposed, thrusting in his tongue and tickling the clitoris with the end of it; and moistening his middle-finger he quickly inserts it into her dark little hum-hole while, forming a two-pronged fork with that finger and the index, he folds hack the other digits and insinuates the latter in the cunt Now all is at work at once, and soon the lady finds herself in heaven and gratefully shoots her soft roe into the mouth of her sucking lover.

2 Selfish Heads and Tails

The man being on his knees leaning backwards, supported by a pile of cushions, the woman comes and places herself upon him, her face on his knees, her belly on his breast her head towards the ground, her arse up in the air, legs and thighs wide open, her feet and knees under the arms of the man, right and left He has thus well within his reach the cunt and arse of the woman, but much higher up than in the description « Sixty-Nine Reversed » (No. 4 Chapter 1, 2nd Section « ante »). The man grasps a bum-cheek with each hand, opens the cunt-lips, parting the hair, thrusting in his tongue and making active play on the clitoris.

He can do the same to the arse-hole, or plunge therein a moistened finger. He feels and slaps the bottom, rummages every-where with his hands, but as it is necessary for the woman to use her hands to sustein her body head downwards she cannot frig her lover. Neither can she suck his prick, because she has to keep her head up so that the blood shall not rush to her brain as it has a tendency to do as a result of this position. Soon a flood of feminine essence fills the nose and mouth of the man, proving the happy effect of this style of lascivious enjoyment.

3 Face Fucking

The man lies at full length on the bed; the woman being on her knees facing his feet, above his shoulders, straddling on his face, the thighs wide open. She leans backwards, one hand on the pillows to support her body. The man's face is thus between the woman's thighs and he gamahuches her with the most voluptuous play of his tongue. He passes one hand between her body and the back of one of her thighs and presses the small of her back to draw her towards him. He forms the fork with index and middle-finger of his other hand, closing the other fingers, and pushes one in the arse-hole and the other in the cunt and shoves them in and out, turning them about in every direction, until he feels two orifices nip and pinch him through the palpitations of lust, and at last an abundant discharge bedews his face and drops into his mouth.

I can think of nothing more to tell you, sweet Maudie, and now you are as knowing as I am in all these libidinous theories. I think it is time to experiment a little practically and then retire to rest in each other's arms.

LOVE AND SECURITY; OF, HOW TO FUCK WITHOUT DANGER OF FECUNDATION

Maud. — My darling, I have yet one more thing to ask you and that is some information and explanation concerning so called secret methods, by which a woman can give herself up to the pleasure of the caresses and embraces of the man she loves without danger of getting in the family way.

Charlie. — Frankly, the best and surest way would be to prove mutual love by caresses, without introduction of the prick in the cunt, for if it goes in ever such a little way, or even if the discharge takes place only just within the outer lips, with some women the greedy orifice has such avidity for spunk, that it can suck up enough to effect the dreaded result of conception. A man, if he really loves the woman he fucks and does not wish to risk getting a child, must feel very sure of the moral control he exercises over himself to get into her with the firm intention to withdraw in time to discharge completely outside. He must he away before the fountain starts playing and not return until the prick be carefully washed and pressed, so that not a drop of seed remains at the end, nor in the canal, which is needless to say the man cleans at once by the simple act of pissing. The least drop into the vagina suffices to cause pregnancy. The same remark applies to the second introduction, where, after having once gone away, discharging outside, the prick goes back without having been cleansed and wiped, with something remaining of the preceding discharge either at the orifice of the gland or in the canal that can penetrate into the sexual organs of the woman by the friction of a fresh venereal act, even before causing a fresh spurt of semen. Therefore we must be out « too soon » so as not to leave « too late ». To finish, the man can use his hand, or his lady's, or migrate to any other part of her frame as may suit, as I have pointed out in all my descriptions of postures without real intromission. Better be outside « too soon » than to run the risk of dropping the little liquid parcel in the dangerous greedy hole and causing an illnees of nine months duration. To conclude my remarks, I can only say that too much prudence can never do any harm, especially as the doctors with all their learning have not yet been able to tell precisely how the female is fecundated. So I shall be excused if I make mistakes in the delicate subject I am now treating, as what I know is from experience only, having no real scientific knowledge to boast of.

1 No Bottom-Fucking Allowed

One of the secrets of not getting the woman with child is, to begin with, not to put the prick in the cunt, and I note a vulgar error which bars even the arse-hole as being too near the genuine aperture! It has also been said that after a first discharge one may fuck as one will, second and later copulation being unable to cause pregnancy. I need hardly stop to point out the inanity of this belief.

2 Snuffing the Candle

Another way which is as good as any with a man who can be reasonable, even while fucking, is to go ahead and enjoy oneself and content our companion in every way possible, as long as we dislodge our tool before the discharge begins, and slip it up to her navel, or jerk it on one side so that the woman can finish us off with her hand far from the cunt and receive in her soft palm the spunk of which she fears the prolific power ». This is called « Snuffing the Candle ».

3 No Mutual Spending Permitted

Another vulgar error consists simply in not « coming » together, that is to say that the woman takes care not to open her sluice-gates until either before or after the mans dew has moistened her rose. The persons who consider this method as infallible declare that conception only takes place when the lovers spend together, their seed mixing at the moment of the mutual ejaculation, and that the least interval between the two jets deprives the mixture of all its virtue and stops fecundation. I do not believe in this system, although admitting that the pleasure in fucking is doubtless greater when the lovers spend together and that the genital organs in such a case are better disposed to receive the germ. But it does not follow that there will be no conception without simultaneous discharges, as proved by the fact of many wives of icy temperament tearing large families without ever having really « spent » « come » or « enjoyed » in the whole course of their conjugal career. Women violated while under the influence of narcotics, or victims of rape without the slightest feeling of pleasure have also been known to bear children.

4 The French Letter

A well-know check is the use of the French letter, name given to a kind of elongated bag or case made of a very thin skin or fine india-rubber. This is slipped over the prick and, being made for the purpose, has the proper shape and length to fit the member, just as the umbrella case fits an umbrella, with the exception that naturally the French letter is only open at the end where the cock goes in. They are blown out before using to see that they are sound and being wetted stick tightly round the shaft and head of the viril organ.

With ease, the man starts fucking as soon as his cock is thus covered up. His seed, instead of spurting into the woman's vagina, is forced to remain inside the sheathy, which is so thin, that neither the man nor the woman can scarcely perceive its presence during the action, which can be consequently carried to a natural end with the same voluptuous pleasure as if there was nothing at all to separate the sexual parts of lover and mistress.

This protecting skin is also worn to prevent contagion and to guard against venereal disease when fucking doubtful women, but being so thin there is always a doubt that it may burst in the thick of the battle, or the friction of cunt and cock may cause a leak, and then the subtle liquid escaping renders its aid a delusion and a snare. Such accidents may happen, but rarely, especially if a good article is bought of a respectable chemist. I have used them often with ladies who feared pregnancy and never found one split. But their use becomes fastidious and troublesome by the care and bother necessary before going into action, and afterwards as they should be renewed at each fresh fuck.

We have seen some lately which are only little round bags fitting over the nut of the prick, fastening under the ridge of the acorn, and I must not forget to tell you that the late Doctor Ricord, the great French venereal specialist, declared that the

French letter was « a cobweb against contagion and a shield against pleasure ».

5 The Spong

Another precaution against pregnancy that I know of is rounded on a scientific truth, which is that to produce conception the seed should be pure and without the least foreign admixture. A drop of any fluid, a little atmospheric air or anything else you can think of, added to the seed, immediately deprives it of all prolific virtue. If we combine this formula with this other necessity for generation — that the man's seminal fluid must penetrate into the woman's womb to fecundate her — we may make her use a little round fine sponge, about the size of a small nut, fastened to a thin silken string about ten or twelve inches long. This sponge is moistened with weak vinegar and water, or any other acid may be used, if sufficiently diluted, and it is then plunged into the cunt, leaving the end of the riband outside, so as to be able to withdraw after coition, in order to rinse it, moisten it again and replace it for a fresh fuck.

It can be easily understood that, by means of the presence of this moistened sponge in the vagina, not only does the man's discharge find an obstacle to prevent it reaching the womb, but even if some drops do manage to get past the sponge, they are mixed with the acidulated water with which the latter is wetted and this admixture is calculated to rob the liquor of its wonderful procreating power, Instead of the sponge a small india-rubber pessary can also be used. They are sold at all chemists and bandage shops, and sometimes soluble pessaries can be purchased for the same use.

6 The Injection

The last and most convenient check to stop large and small families is that the woman should jump up immediately the man has spent freely within and pump a sufficient quantity of weak vinegar and water into her cunt. I think that this means is certainly as good as any other, but how can the woman tell if the boiling viril essence has not already reached her worn may inject as long as she likes and clean out her vagina and the neck of the womb with oceans of liquid from her enema, but if the tiniest drop of dangerous seed is already within, there is no hope for her.

But all said and done this is a very uncertain and

risky matter, as once the seed is sown it is well-nigh impossible to prevent the child being born, unless criminal practices are resorted to, to the imminent danger of the mother's life.

How many poor girls suffer, if they are a few days behind with their monthly derangement and what relief when the crimson flow appears! And even that means nothing sometimes, as pregnant women often have regular or irregular courses.

I have now told you the little I know to prevent conception. Now let lovers choose and invent fresh means if possible, if they have no confidence in the saying that in love and war many blows are given in vain and the biggest cowards are the soonest captured. Having put on one side, as I told you, all religious scruples when treating of these matters, I have great indulgence for the weaknesses of women who wish for pleasure without running the risk of getting with child. But this indulgence I no longer grant when I hear a proposition to destroy the result of their voluptuousness, as in that case a sin is committed against society at large. The act which was the original cause can no longer be excused and becomes nothing more than the first step in the path of crime. When checks are employed to prevent conception, no harm is done;

we are no more guilty than when we formicate each other, but if you seek to destroy the generative result you murder a being who belongs to the community of which you yourself are a member, and you trample under foot all human and social laws.

So I shall tell nothing concerning the methods in vogue to procure abortion, which means, as you know, the destruction of a child already conceived and breathing.

Maud. — And you are right, this last topic is so horrible to my mind that it does not inspire me with the least curiosity. I cannot thank you enough for all your teaching, being now fully satisfied on all the obseure points that I wished cleared up, and I am ready to prove my gratitude in any way you like for the trouble you have taken and the patience and amiability you have shown.

CONCLUSION

(Here the dialogue ceases. The lovers give themselves up to lewd and libidinous voluptuous enjoyment more enjoyable than any talk, and sleep overcomes them in each other's arms, until the moment arrives for separation and Maud starts off to the country to effect her alibi).

FINIS

CPSIA information can be obtained
at www.ICGtesting.com
Printed in the USA
FSOW01n1521181216
28729FS

9 780994 295514